DIABETIC-FRIENDLY MEAL PLANS FOR WEIGHT LOSS

Affordable Strategies for Effective Weight Management and Wellness

JAMES HOFFMAN

Table of Contents

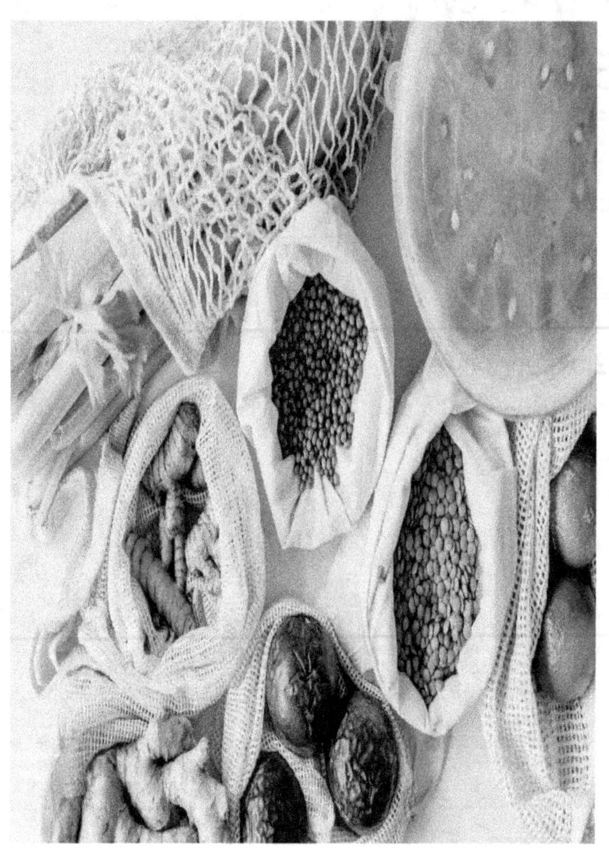

INTRODUCTION

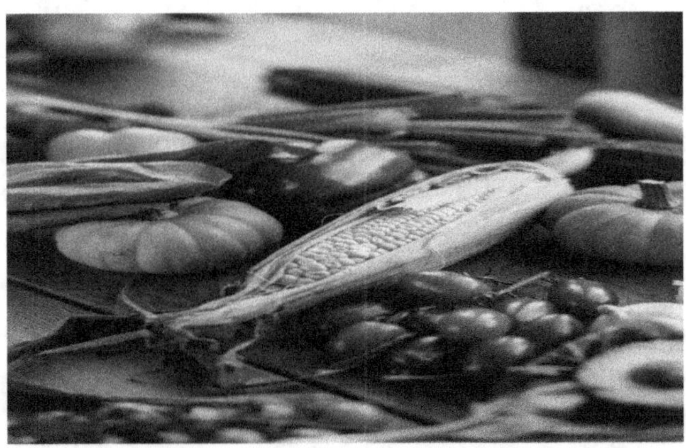

Understanding Diabetes and Weight Loss
The prevalence of diabetes has reached alarming proportions globally, heralding a critical intersection between this chronic condition and the realm of weight management. According to the World Health Organization (WHO), an estimated 422 million people were living with diabetes worldwide as of January 2022. This number is anticipated to rise, driven by factors such as sedentary lifestyles, unhealthy diets, and an aging population.

The link between diabetes and weight management is intricate and bidirectional. Excess body weight, particularly abdominal obesity, is a well-established risk factor for the development of Type 2 diabetes. The adipose tissue, especially in the abdominal area, contributes to insulin resistance, where the body's cells become less responsive to insulin. This resistance, coupled with impaired insulin production, characterizes the pathophysiology of Type 2 diabetes.

Conversely, diabetes itself can present challenges to weight management. Insulin, a key hormone in blood sugar regulation, plays a role in fat storage. In conditions of insulin resistance or deficiency, the body may struggle to efficiently utilize glucose for energy, leading to increased fat storage and potential weight gain.
The delicate balance required for effective weight management in individuals with diabetes involves addressing both sides of this equation. Lifestyle modifications, including dietary changes and increased physical activity, play a crucial role. A well-structured weight management plan for those with diabetes not only aims to achieve a healthy weight but also prioritizes stable blood sugar control, improved insulin sensitivity, and overall cardiovascular health.

In essence, the prevalence of diabetes underscores the urgency of integrating weight management strategies into public health initiatives. Understanding the dynamic relationship between diabetes and weight is essential for crafting holistic interventions that not only address the rising prevalence of diabetes but also promote sustainable and effective weight management for those affected.

Importance of Diabetic-Friendly Meal Plans
Creating meal plans tailored to the specific needs of individuals with diabetes is not merely a dietary preference; it is a crucial component in managing this chronic condition effectively. The significance of such personalized meal planning extends to various aspects that directly impact overall health and well-being.

- Tailoring meal plans ensures a balanced distribution of carbohydrates, helping manage blood sugar levels effectively.

- A well-designed meal plan considers the balance of macronutrients, aiding in improved insulin sensitivity.

- Personalized meal plans facilitate portion control, aiding in calorie management crucial for weight loss or maintenance.

- Tailored meal plan can accommodate individual dietary preferences and cultural influences, enhancing adherence.

- Personalized meal plans serve as educational tools, empowering individuals with the knowledge to make informed food choices.

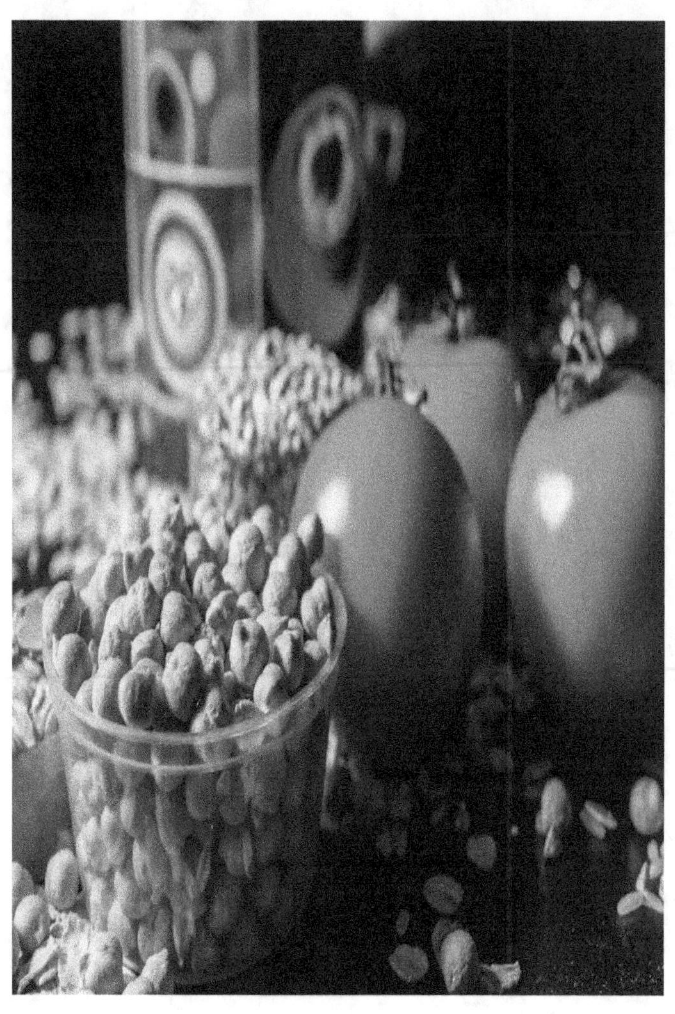

CHAPTER ONE

Basics of Diabetes and Nutrition

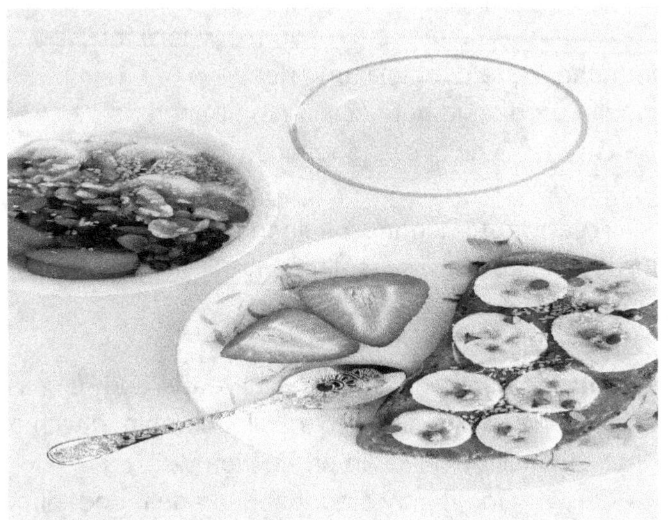

Overview of Diabetes Types

Diabetes is a complex group of metabolic disorders characterized by elevated blood sugar levels. There are several types of diabetes, each with distinct causes, characteristics, and management approaches. Understanding the distinctions between the different types of diabetes is crucial for appropriate diagnosis, treatment, and management strategies. Each type requires a tailored approach, considering the unique characteristics and contributing factors associated with the specific form of diabetes. Regular monitoring, lifestyle adjustments, and medical guidance play integral roles in managing diabetes effectively. The main types:

1. **Type 1 Diabetes**
  - **Cause:** Autoimmune response where the immune system attacks and destroys insulin-producing beta cells in the pancreas.
  - **Onset:** Typically diagnosed in childhood or adolescence.
  - **Treatment:** Requires lifelong insulin therapy through injections or insulin pump.

2. **Type 2 Diabetes**:
  - **Cause:** Insulin resistance, where the body's cells don't respond effectively to insulin, combined with a gradual decline in insulin production.
  - **Onset:** Commonly diagnosed in adulthood, but increasingly seen in younger individuals.
  - **Treatment:** Managed through lifestyle modifications, oral medications, and, in some cases, insulin therapy.

3. **Gestational Diabetes:**
  - **Cause:** Develops during pregnancy when the body cannot produce enough insulin to meet increased demands.
  - **Onset:** Typically diagnosed during the second or third trimester.

- **Treatment:** Managed through dietary changes, exercise, and sometimes medication; often resolves after childbirth.

4. **Prediabetes:**
   - **Condition:** Blood sugar levels higher than normal but not yet in the diabetes range.
   - **Risk:** Increases the risk of developing Type 2 diabetes and cardiovascular diseases.
   - **Prevention:** Lifestyle changes can often reverse prediabetes.

5. **Monogenic Diabetes:**
   - **Cause:** Caused by a mutation in a single gene, leading to impaired insulin production.
   - **Onset:** Can occur at any age, often in adolescence or early adulthood.
   - **Treatment:** Varied, depending on the specific genetic mutation; may include oral medications or insulin.

6. **Secondary Diabetes:**
   - **Cause:** Develops as a result of another medical condition, such as pancreatic diseases or certain medications.
   - **Onset:** Variable, depends on the underlying cause.
   - **Treatment:** Managing the underlying condition often helps control blood sugar levels.

Role of Nutrition in Diabetes Management

The crucial role of nutrition in managing diabetes cannot be overstated; it serves as a cornerstone in achieving optimal blood sugar control, overall health, and preventing complications. Nutrition in essence is a cornerstone in diabetes management, influencing various facets of the condition, from blood sugar control and insulin sensitivity to weight management and overall health. A thoughtful and individualized approach to nutrition is fundamental for empowering individuals with diabetes to make sustainable, health-promoting choices and lead fulfilling lives. The key aspects highlighting the significance of nutrition in diabetes management are:

1. **Blood Sugar Control:**
   - **Carbohydrate Management:** Nutrition influences blood sugar levels directly through the management of carbohydrate intake. Understanding the impact of different carbohydrates helps in regulating blood sugar.
   - **Meal Timing:** Consistent meal timing and spacing contribute to stable blood sugar levels throughout the day.

2. **Insulin Sensitivity:**
   - **Nutrient-Dense Choices:** Opting for nutrient-dense foods supports insulin sensitivity, helping the body utilize insulin more effectively.

  - **Balanced Macronutrients:** Proper balance of carbohydrates, proteins, and fats in meals contributes to improved insulin function.

3. Weight Management:
  - **Caloric Balance:** Nutrition plays a key role in achieving and maintaining a healthy weight, crucial for managing insulin resistance and reducing the risk of complications.
  - **Healthy Food Choices:** Emphasizing whole, unprocessed foods aids in weight management without compromising essential nutrients.

4. Heart Health:
  - **Reducing Saturated Fats:** Nutrition influences heart health by promoting choices low in saturated and trans fats, reducing the risk of cardiovascular complications associated with diabetes.
  - **Incorporating Heart-Healthy Foods:** Including foods rich in omega-3 fatty acids, fiber, and antioxidants supports cardiovascular well-being.

5. Preventing Complications:
  - **Sodium Control:** Managing sodium intake is essential to prevent complications such as high blood pressure and kidney issues often associated with diabetes.
  - **Nutrient Diversity:** A diverse and balanced diet helps prevent nutrient deficiencies, promoting overall health and reducing the risk of complications.

6. **Individualized Approach:**
  - **Personalized Plans:** Tailoring nutrition plans to individual preferences, cultural influences, and specific health needs enhances adherence and promotes long-term success.
  - **Consistent Adherence:** Individualized plans increase the likelihood of consistent adherence to dietary recommendations.

7. **Education and Empowerment:**
  - **Understanding Food Labels:** Nutrition education empowers individuals to make informed choices by understanding food labels and selecting appropriate options.
  - **Meal Planning Skills:** Developing skills in meal planning and preparation fosters a sense of control and self-efficacy in managing diabetes through nutrition.

8. **Stress Reduction:**
  - **Balancing Macronutrients:** A well-balanced diet helps stabilize energy levels, contributing to stress reduction, which is crucial for managing blood sugar levels.

9. **Preventing Hypoglycemia:**
  - **Balancing Meals and Snacks:** Strategic meal planning helps prevent hypoglycemia by avoiding prolonged periods without food and maintaining consistent nutrient intake.

Carbohydrates, Proteins, and Fats: Balancing Nutrients

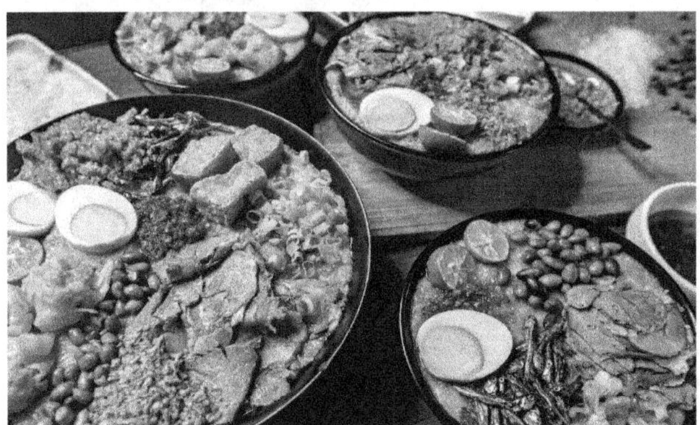

Balancing carbohydrates, proteins, and fats is a fundamental aspect of managing diabetes, as it directly influences blood sugar levels, insulin sensitivity, and overall health. Let's take a closer look at how to achieve a balanced approach to these macronutrients:

1. **Carbohydrates:**
   - **Focus on Quality:** Choose complex carbohydrates with a low glycemic index, such as whole grains, legumes, and vegetables. These release glucose into the bloodstream more slowly, avoiding rapid spikes in blood sugar.
   - **Portion Control:** Monitor portion sizes to regulate carbohydrate intake. Pay attention to total carbohydrates per serving and spread them evenly throughout meals and snacks.

- **Timing Matters:** Distribute carbohydrate intake evenly throughout the day to prevent large fluctuations in blood sugar levels. Consider consuming carbohydrates before or after physical activity.

2. **Proteins:**
   - **Lean Protein Sources:** Opt for lean protein sources such as poultry, fish, tofu, legumes, and low-fat dairy. These offer vital nutrients without excessive saturated fats.
   - **Portion Moderation:** Control portion sizes to avoid overconsumption of proteins, as excessive intake can contribute to increased calorie and fat intake.
   - **Balanced Meals:** Include a source of lean protein in each meal to promote satiety and stabilize blood sugar levels.

3. **Fats:**
   - **Healthy Fats:** Emphasize sources of healthy fats, including avocados, nuts, seeds, and olive oil. These fats have cardiovascular benefits and can contribute to overall health.
   - **Limit Saturated and Trans Fats:** Minimize the intake of saturated and trans fats, commonly found in fried foods, processed snacks, and certain animal products. These fats can contribute to insulin resistance and heart health issues.
   - **Portion Awareness:** Be mindful of portion sizes, as fats are calorie-dense. Incorporate them

in appropriate amounts to support nutrient absorption and maintain a healthy weight.

4. **Balancing the Plate:**
- **Plate Method:** Use the plate method to create well-balanced meals. Fill half your plate with non-starchy vegetables, a quarter with lean protein, and a quarter with whole grains or starchy vegetables.
- **Snack Planning:** Apply similar principles to snacks, combining a protein source with a small portion of carbohydrates for sustained energy.

5. **Monitoring and Adjusting:**
- **Blood Sugar Monitoring:** Regularly monitor blood sugar levels to observe the impact of different macronutrient ratios on glycemic control.
- **Individualized Approach:** Adjust nutrient balance based on individual responses, considering factors like medication, physical activity, and personal preferences.

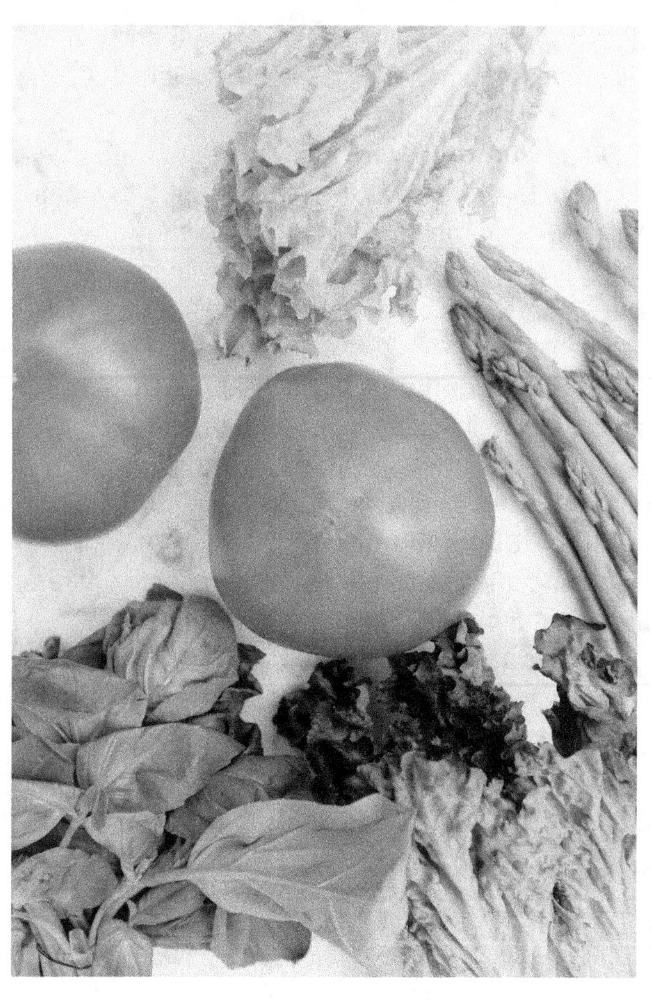

CHAPTER TWO

Setting Weight Loss Goals for Diabetics

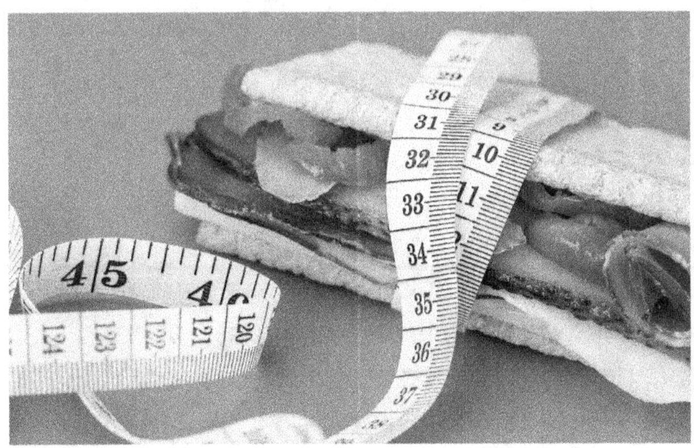

Healthy Weight Goals for Diabetics

Healthy weight goals for individuals with diabetes are personalized targets that aim to achieve and maintain an optimal body weight to enhance overall health and manage the condition effectively. These goals take into account individual characteristics, such as age, height, activity level, and any existing health conditions. Let us explore some key considerations when defining healthy weight goals for individuals with diabetes:

1. **Body Mass Index (BMI):**
   - **Reference Point:** BMI is a commonly used tool to assess body weight in relation to height. A BMI within the normal range (18.5 to 24.9) is generally considered a healthy goal.
   - **Individual Variations:** Recognize that BMI has limitations and may not account for variations in muscle mass. It is crucial to consider overall health and body composition.

2. **Weight Loss Targets:**
   - **Gradual Approach:** Aim for gradual and sustainable weight loss, typically around 1-2 pounds per week. Rapid weight loss can be associated with muscle loss and may not be maintainable in the long term.
   - **Total Percentage:** Aiming for a weight loss of 5-10% of total body weight is often associated with improvements in insulin sensitivity and overall diabetes management.

3. **Waist Circumference:**
   - **Abdominal Fat Considerations:** Waist circumference is an indicator of abdominal fat, which is particularly relevant for individuals with diabetes. A healthy waist circumference is generally considered less than 35 inches for women and 40 inches for men.
   - **Heart Health**: Reduction in abdominal fat can contribute to improved insulin sensitivity and heart health.

4. **Individual Health Status:**
   - **Comorbid Conditions:** Consider any existing health conditions, such as cardiovascular disease or hypertension, which may influence weight goals.
   - **Medication Impact:** Some diabetes medications can affect weight, so adjustments may be necessary to align with overall health goals.

5. **Lifestyle Factors:**
   - **Physical Activity:** Integrate regular physical activity into the plan, as exercise not only contributes to weight management but also improves insulin sensitivity and overall well-being.
   - **Dietary Patterns:** Focus on a balanced and nutrient-dense diet that supports weight goals and meets the nutritional needs of individuals with diabetes.

6. **Collaboration with Healthcare Professionals:**
   - **Individualized Plans:** Work closely with healthcare professionals, including dietitians and physicians, to create individualized weight management plans.
   - **Monitoring and Adjusting:** Regularly monitor progress and adjust goals as needed based on individual responses and changing health conditions.

Creating Realistic Targets

Creating achievable and realistic weight loss targets is essential for long-term success and overall well-being. ***It's a journey that involves patience, consistency, and a positive mindset.*** Guide to help set realistic and attainable weight loss goals:

1. **Understand Your Starting Point:**
   - **Assess Current Weight:** Begin by understanding your current weight and body mass index (BMI).
   - **Consider Health Factors:** Take into account any existing health conditions, medications, and lifestyle factors that may influence weight loss.
2. **Set Incremental Goals:**
   - **Gradual Approach:** Aim for gradual weight loss, typically 1-2 pounds per week. Rapid weight loss is often unsustainable and may not promote long-term success.
   - **Total Percentage:** Consider setting initial goals to lose 5-10% of your current body weight. This is associated with health improvements and is an achievable target.

3. **Consider Your Lifestyle:**
   - **Assess Daily Habits:** Evaluate your current lifestyle, including dietary patterns and physical activity levels. Identify small, realistic changes that can be incorporated into your routine.

   - **Realistic Adjustments:** Set goals that align with your daily life, considering work, family commitments, and other responsibilities.

4. Be Specific and Measurable:
   - **Define Clear Goals:** Clearly define your weight loss goals. For example, instead of a vague goal like "lose weight," specify "lose 10 pounds in 8 weeks."
   - **Use Metrics:** Incorporate measurable metrics, such as pounds lost, waist circumference reduction, or changes in clothing size.

5. Focus on Behavioral Changes:
   - **Identify Habits to Change:** Pinpoint specific behaviors contributing to weight gain, such as unhealthy eating patterns or sedentary habits.
   - **Set Behavioral Goals:** Establish goals centered around changing these behaviors. For instance, aim to include more vegetables in meals or increase daily steps.

6. Include Non-Scale Victories:
   - **Broader Indicators:** Recognize achievements beyond the scale, such as increased energy levels, improved sleep, or enhanced mood.
   - **Celebrate Milestones:** Celebrate non-scale victories to maintain motivation and reinforce positive changes.

7. Involve Professional Guidance:

- **Consult Healthcare Professionals:** Seek guidance from healthcare professionals, including dietitians or nutritionists, to develop a personalized plan.
- **Regular Check-Ins:** Schedule regular check-ins with professionals to monitor progress, receive support, and make adjustments if needed.

8. Set Realistic Timelines:

- **Consider Long-Term Goals:** Understand that sustainable weight loss is a long-term journey. Set realistic timelines for achieving your goals, keeping in mind that slow and steady progress is key.
- **Adapt as Needed:** Be flexible and willing to adapt goals based on your body's response and changing circumstances.

9. Build a Support System:

- **Involve Friends and Family:** Share your goals with supportive friends or family members who can provide encouragement.
- **Join a Support Group:** Consider joining a weight loss or fitness community for additional motivation and shared experiences.

10. Celebrate Achievements:

- **Acknowledge Progress:** Celebrate your achievements, both big and small.
- **Learn from Setbacks:** Recognize that setbacks may occur. Learn from them, adjust your approach

if needed, and continue working towards your goals.

Monitoring Progress

Below is a tabular representation of how to monitor progress in weight loss in a diabetic-friendly context:

Monitoring Method	Description
Weighing Scale	- Weigh regularly, using the same scale and conditions.
	- Focus on overall trends rather than daily fluctuations.
Body Measurements	- Measure waist, hips, and chest regularly using a tape measure.
	- Reductions in these measurements may indicate fat loss.
Progress Photos	- Take full-body photos at consistent intervals (e.g., monthly).
	- Capture front, side, and back views for a

	comprehensive view.
Clothing Fit	- Pay attention to changes in how clothes fit, indicating progress.
	- Try on a designated "goal" piece of clothing periodically.
Physical Fitness	- Monitor improvements in strength, endurance, and fitness milestones.
	- Track changes in workout intensity, duration, or weights lifted.
Energy Levels	- Observe changes in energy levels as an indicator of improved well-being.
	- Pay attention to mood and sleep quality improvements.
Nutritional Habits	- Keep a food journal to track meals and identify patterns.
	- Practice mindful eating, paying attention to hunger and fullness cues.
Support System	- Share goals with an accountability partner for

	regular check-ins.
	- Join diabetic-friendly weight loss communities for support.
Celebrate Achievements	- Acknowledge and celebrate small milestones and non-scale victories.
	- Positive reinforcement is crucial for maintaining motivation.
Professional Guidance	- Regularly consult with healthcare professionals for personalized advice. - Ensure that weight loss goals align with diabetes management.

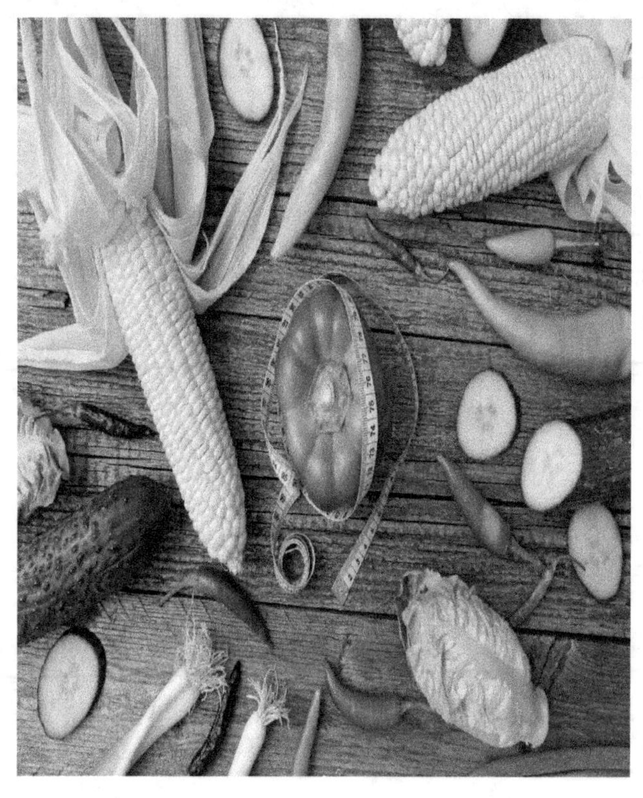

CHAPTER THREE

Diabetic-Friendly Foods for Weight Loss

Low-Glycemic Index Foods

Low-glycemic index (GI) foods have a slower impact on blood sugar levels, making them beneficial for individuals, especially those with diabetes, as they help maintain more stable glucose levels. Hereunder are examples of GI foods:

Food Category	Low-GI Foods
Grains and Cereals	- Quinoa - Barley - Bulgur - Whole grain pasta - Oats - Brown rice
Legumes	- Chickpeas - Lentils - Kidney beans - Black beans - Green peas
Fruits	- Cherries

	- Apples - Pears - Plums - Berries (strawberries, blueberries, raspberries) - Grapefruit
Vegetables	- Broccoli - Cauliflower - Spinach - Kale - Tomatoes - Zucchini
Dairy and Alternatives	- Greek yogurt (unsweetened) - Milk (preferably low-fat or non-fat)
Nuts and Seeds	- Peanuts - Almonds - Walnuts - Chia seeds - Flaxseeds
Snacks and Sweets	- Dark chocolate (in moderation) - Hummus - Guacamole
Beverages	- Unsweetened almond milk - Herbal tea - Water

Incorporating Fiber in the Diet

Incorporating a variety of fiber-rich choices into your diet can contribute to better digestion, help maintain a healthy weight, improve blood sugar control and support overall well-being. Remember to drink plenty of water when increasing your fiber intake.

Examples of fiber-rich foods are Whole grains (Brown rice, Quinoa, Oats), Legumes (Lentils, Chickpeas, Black beans, Kidney beans), Fruits (Apples with skin, Berries, Pears, Oranges), Vegetables (Broccoli, Spinach, Brussels sprouts, Carrots) Nuts and Seeds (Almonds, Chia seeds, Flaxseeds, Sunflower seeds) Root Vegetables (Sweet potatoes, Beets, Turnips).

Benefits of Fiber-Rich Choices:

1. **Blood Sugar Regulation:**

   - <u>Stabilizes Glucose Levels:</u> Fiber slows the absorption of sugar, preventing rapid spikes in blood sugar levels after meals.

   - <u>Improved Insulin Sensitivity:</u> Regular consumption of fiber has been associated with enhanced insulin sensitivity.

2. **Satiety and Weight Management:**

   - <u>Enhanced Fullness:</u> High-fiber foods promote a feeling of fullness, reducing overall food intake and supporting weight management.

   - <u>Calorie Dilution:</u> Many fiber-rich foods are low in calories, allowing for larger portions without excess calorie intake.

3. **Digestive Health:**
   - <u>Prevents Constipation:</u> Fiber adds bulk to stool, promoting regular bowel movements and preventing constipation.
   - <u>Supports Gut Microbiota:</u> Certain fibers are prebiotic, nourishing beneficial gut bacteria and supporting a healthy microbiome.

4. **Heart Health:**
   - <u>Lowers Cholesterol:</u> Soluble fiber, found in foods like oats and legumes, can help lower LDL cholesterol levels, promoting heart health.
   - <u>Blood Pressure Regulation:</u> Some fibers contribute to maintaining healthy blood pressure levels.

5. **Blood Lipid Management:**
   - <u>Regulates Triglycerides:</u> Certain fibers have been shown to help regulate triglyceride levels in the blood.

General Tips for Diabetic-Friendly Choices

- **Whole Foods Emphasis:**Opt for whole, minimally processed sources of fiber and lean protein.

- **Diverse Sources:** Include a variety of fiber-rich foods (vegetables, fruits, whole grains) and lean protein sources (poultry, fish, legumes, tofu).
- **Portion Control:** Be mindful of portion sizes to maintain a balanced diet without excessive calorie intake.
- **Hydration:** Adequate water intake is essential, especially when increasing fiber intake.

Choosing Lean Proteins

Choosing lean proteins is important for maintaining a healthy and well-balanced diet, especially for individuals with diabetes. Remember that a well-rounded diet includes a mix of protein sources to provide essential amino acids and a variety of nutrients. Let's explore some guidelines for selecting lean protein sources:

1. **Poultry:**
   - <u>Skinless Chicken:</u> Opt for skinless chicken breasts or thighs, as removing the skin reduces saturated fat content.
   - <u>Turkey:</u> Choose lean cuts of turkey, and consider ground turkey with lower fat percentages.

2. **Fish:**
   - <u>Fatty Fish:</u> Include omega-3-rich fish like salmon, mackerel, and trout, as they offer heart-healthy fats.
   - <u>White Fish:</u> Options such as cod, haddock, and flounder are lower in fat and calories.

3. **Lean Cuts of Meat:**
   - <u>Lean Beef:</u> Choose lean cuts like sirloin, tenderloin, or round cuts. Look for the terms "loin" or "round" when buying beef.
   - <u>Pork:</u> Opt for loin or tenderloin cuts of pork, and trim visible fat.

4. **Plant-Based Proteins:**
   - <u>Legumes:</u> Include beans, lentils, and chickpeas as excellent plant-based protein sources.
   - <u>Tofu and Tempeh:</u> Incorporate tofu and tempeh, which are rich in protein and versatile in recipes.

5. **Eggs:**
   - <u>Egg Whites:</u> Choose egg whites or a mix of whole eggs and egg whites to reduce overall fat and cholesterol intake.
   - <u>Omega-3 Enriched Eggs:</u> Consider eggs enriched with omega-3 for additional heart-healthy benefits.

6. **Low-Fat Dairy:**
   - <u>Greek Yogurt:</u> Opt for plain, non-fat or low-fat Greek yogurt, which is rich in protein.
   - <u>Skim Milk:</u> Choose skim or low-fat milk for a protein-rich, calcium source.

7. **Processed and Cured Meats:**
   - <u>Minimize Processed Meats:</u> Limit consumption of processed and cured meats, such as sausages and bacon, as they can be high in saturated fats and sodium.

8. **Preparation Methods:**

   - <u>Grilling and Baking:</u> Use grilling, baking, steaming, or broiling methods to cook proteins without adding excess fats.

   - <u>Avoid Frying:</u> Minimize frying or use healthier frying techniques, such as air frying with minimal oil.

9. **Portion Control:**

   - <u>Mindful Portions:</u> Be mindful of portion sizes to avoid excessive calorie intake. Aim for a balance between protein, carbohydrates, and fats.

10. **Label Reading:**

   - <u>Check Nutrition Labels:</u> When buying packaged proteins, check nutrition labels for fat content, especially saturated fat and trans fat.

   - <u>Choose Unprocessed Options:</u> Opt for minimally processed or unprocessed protein sources.

11. **Hydration:**

   - <u>Stay Hydrated:</u> Adequate hydration supports overall health and digestion, especially when consuming protein-rich foods.

The benefits of incorporating lean proteins into your diet include:

1. Blood Sugar Control:

   - <u>Slow Release of Amino Acids:</u> Lean proteins are digested more slowly, leading to a gradual release of amino acids and preventing rapid increases in blood sugar.

   - <u>Insulin Sensitivity:</u> Adequate protein intake supports insulin sensitivity.

2. **Satiety and Weight Management:**

   - <u>Appetite Control:</u> Protein-rich meals induce a greater feeling of fullness, reducing overall calorie consumption.

   - <u>Preservation of Lean Body Mass:</u> Adequate protein intake supports muscle maintenance during weight loss.

3. **Muscle Health:**

   - <u>Muscle Repair and Growth:</u> Proteins are essential for muscle repair and growth, especially important for individuals engaging in physical activity.

   - <u>Metabolic Rate:</u> The thermic effect of protein contributes to a higher metabolic rate, supporting weight management.

4. **Cardiovascular Health:**

   - <u>Reduced Saturated Fats:</u> Lean protein sources often contain lower levels of saturated fats, promoting heart health.

   - <u>Cholesterol Management:</u> Some lean proteins, such as fish, contribute to favorable cholesterol profiles.

5. **Nutrient Density:**

  - <u>Rich in Essential Nutrients:</u> Lean proteins are often rich in essential nutrients, including vitamins and minerals.

  - <u>Balanced Diet:</u> Inclusion of lean proteins ensures a balanced macronutrient profile in the diet.

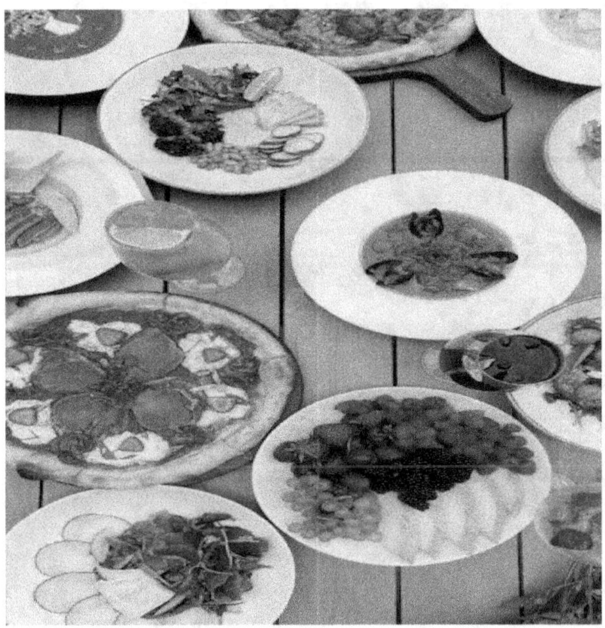

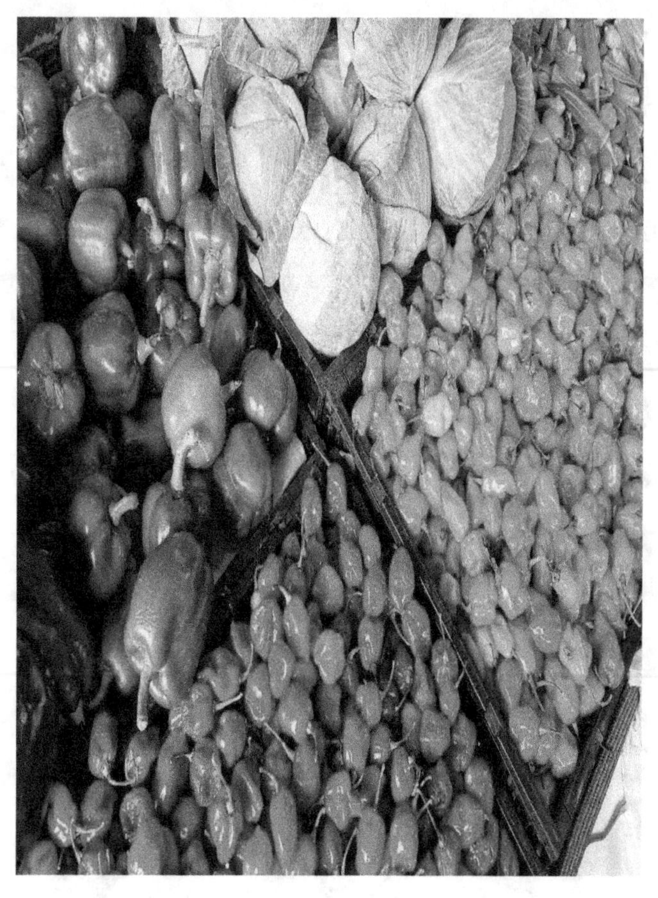

CHAPTER FOUR

Crafting Balanced and Nutrient-Rich Meals

Sample Diabetic-Friendly Meal Plans

Below are two sample meal plans catering to individuals with diabetes. These plans focus on a balanced intake of carbohydrates, lean proteins, healthy fats, and fiber to help manage blood sugar levels. Please note that these are general examples, and individual nutritional needs may vary. Portion sizes and specific food choices can be adjusted based on individual preferences, nutritional needs, and any recommendations from healthcare professionals.

Sample Meal Plan 1:

Meal	Food Choices
Breakfast	- Scrambled eggs with spinach and tomatoes - Whole-grain toast - Greek yogurt with fresh berries
Mid-Morning Snack	- Handful of almonds or walnuts - Apple slices

Lunch	- Grilled chicken breast or tofu salad with mixed greens, cherry tomatoes, and vinaigrette dressing - Quinoa or brown rice on the side
Afternoon Snack	- Carrot and cucumber sticks with hummus
Dinner	- Baked salmon or lentil stew - Steamed broccoli and cauliflower - Quinoa or wild rice
Evening Snack	- Low-fat cottage cheese with a small pear

Sample Meal Plan 2:

Meal	Food Choices
Breakfast	- Overnight oats made with rolled oats, chia seeds, almond milk, topped with sliced strawberries and a sprinkle of nuts
Mid-Morning Snack	- A small banana with a tablespoon of peanut

	butter
Lunch	- Turkey or veggie wrap with whole-grain tortilla, lean turkey slices or plant-based protein, lettuce, tomatoes, and mustard - Mixed green salad
Afternoon Snack	- Non-fat Greek yogurt with a handful of blueberries
Dinner	- Stir-fried tofu or grilled chicken with colorful vegetables (bell peppers, broccoli, snap peas) in a light soy sauce - Quinoa or cauliflower rice
Evening Snack	- Sliced cucumber and cherry tomatoes with a drizzle of olive oil and a pinch of salt

Notes:

Portion Control: Be mindful of serving sizes to regulate calorie intake.

Hydration: Ensure adequate water intake throughout the day.

Regular Monitoring: Monitor blood sugar levels regularly and adjust the meal plan as needed.

Individual Variations: Adjust the meal plans based on personal preferences, nutritional needs, and any specific dietary recommendations from healthcare professionals.

Portion Control Strategies

Effective portion control is essential for managing weight, blood sugar levels, and overall health, especially for individuals with diabetes. Portion control is not about deprivation but about making mindful choices that support overall health and well-being. It's crucial to individualize these strategies based on personal preferences and nutritional needs.

Some workable strategies to help control portions:

1. **Use Smaller Plates and Bowls:**
   - Opt for smaller dishware to create the illusion of larger portions. This can help with portion perception and prevent overeating.

2. **Practice Mindful Eating:**
   - Eat slowly and savor each bite. Pay attention to the flavors, textures, and sensations of the food. Mindful eating allows you to recognize fullness cues, preventing overconsumption.

3. **Divide Your Plate:**

   - Use the plate method to visualize portion sizes: Fill half your plate with non-starchy vegetables, one-quarter with lean protein, and one-quarter with whole grains or starchy vegetables.

4. **Pre-Portion Snacks:**

   - Divide snacks into single-serving portions to avoid mindless munching. This can be especially helpful with items like nuts or chips.

5. **Read Nutrition Labels:**

   - Check serving sizes on nutrition labels. Pay attention to portion sizes, and be mindful of the number of servings in a package.

6. **Use Measuring Tools:**

   - Utilize measuring cups, spoons, or a kitchen scale to portion out food accurately. This helps you become familiar with appropriate serving sizes.

7. **Listen to Hunger and Fullness Signals:**

   - Pay attention to your body's hunger and fullness cues. Eat when you feel hungry and stop when you reach a satisfying level of fullness. Avoid eating out of boredom or emotional reasons.

8. **Plan Meals and Snacks:**

- Prearrange meals and snacks to prevent spontaneous eating. Having a structured eating schedule can help control portion sizes and maintain stable blood sugar levels.

9. **Avoid Eating Directly from Packages:**
   - Portion out your food onto a plate rather than eating directly from a bag or box. This helps prevent mindless eating and encourages awareness of portion sizes.

10. **Understand Portion Size Guidelines:**
    - Familiarize yourself with general portion size guidelines. For example, a serving of lean protein is typically around 3 ounces, a serving of grains is about ½ cup, and a serving of vegetables is one cup.

11. **Limit Liquid Calories:**
    - Be mindful of liquid calories, including sugary beverages and alcoholic drinks. Opt for water, herbal tea, or other low-calorie, sugar-free options.

12. **Be Cautious at Restaurants:**
    - Share entrees or ask for a to-go box at the beginning of the meal to set aside a portion. Restaurants often serve larger portions than needed.

13. **Track Your Food Intake:**

- Utilize a food journal or a mobile application to monitor your meals.This helps create awareness of what and how much you're eating.

14. Learn Portion Estimation:
- Develop the ability to estimate portion sizes visually. For instance, a portion of meat is approximately equivalent to the dimensions of a deck of cards.

15. Be Flexible with Treats:
- Indulge in occasional treats, but remain conscious of portion sizes. Savor the flavors without overindulging.

Meal Timing for Stable Blood Sugar

Meal timing plays a crucial role in managing stable blood sugar levels, especially for individuals with diabetes.Effective meal timing is a component of overall diabetes management. Regular monitoring and adjustments will help maintain stable blood sugar levels throughout the day. Guidelines to consider for effective meal timing:

1. Regular Meal Schedule:
- Aim for consistent meal times each day. Establishing a routine helps regulate blood sugar levels and supports medication or insulin schedules.

2. **Balanced Meals:**
   - Include a balance of carbohydrates, proteins, and healthy fats in each meal. This helps slow down the absorption of glucose, preventing rapid spikes in blood sugar.

3. **Spacing Meals:**
   - Space meals evenly throughout the day. This typically involves having three main meals and incorporating healthy snacks between if needed. Avoid long periods without eating.

4. **Consider Glycemic Index:**
   - Choose carbohydrates with a lower glycemic index (GI). Low-GI foods are digested more slowly, leading to a gradual rise in blood sugar.

5. **Pre-Meal Blood Sugar Checks:**
   - Check your blood sugar levels before meals to understand your baseline. This information can guide food choices and portion sizes.

6. **Pre-Exercise Snack:**
   - If engaging in physical activity, consider having a small, balanced snack before exercise to prevent low blood sugar levels.

7. **Post-Exercise Meals:**
   - Consume a balanced meal or snack after exercising to replenish energy stores. This is particularly important for individuals on medications that may cause hypoglycemia.

8. **Bedtime Snack:**
   - Some individuals may benefit from a small, balanced snack before bedtime to prevent nocturnal hypoglycemia. Consult with healthcare professionals for personalized advice.

9. **Avoid Late-Night Heavy Meals:**
   - Try to finish eating at least a few hours before bedtime. Late-night heavy meals can impact blood sugar levels and may interfere with sleep.

10. **Hydration:**
   - Stay hydrated throughout the day. Water is essential for overall health and can help control hunger, preventing overeating.

11. **Adjust Meal Timing with Medications:**
   - Align meal timing with medication schedules. Some medications may require adjustments based on when you eat.

12. **Listen to Your Body:**
   - Pay attention to hunger and fullness cues. Eat when hungry and stop when satisfied.

13. **Consult with Healthcare Professionals:**
   - Work closely with your healthcare team, including a registered dietitian and your healthcare provider, to tailor meal timing to your specific needs.

14. **Monitor Blood Sugar Levels:**

- Regularly monitor blood sugar levels to
understand how different meals and meal timings
affect your readings. Adjust your meal plan
accordingly.

15. **Individualized Approach:**
- Recognize that individual responses to meal
timing can vary. What works for one person may
not work for another. Personalize your approach
based on your lifestyle and preferences.

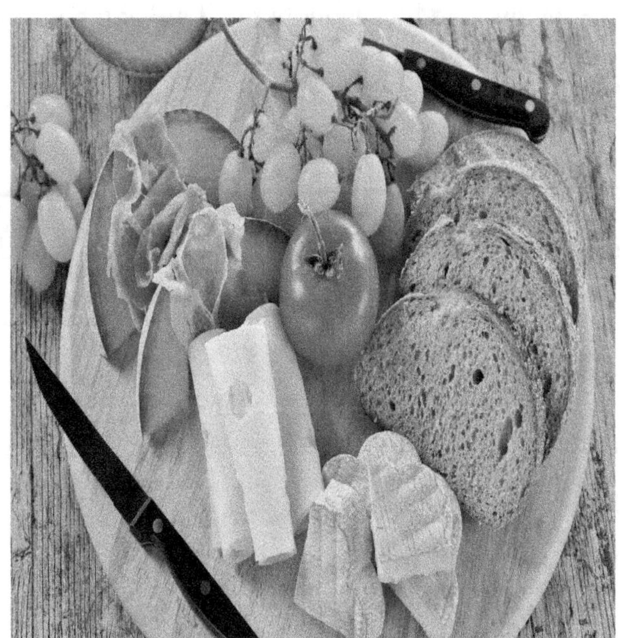

CHAPTER 5

Meal Prep and Planning

Importance of Meal Planning for Diabetics

Meal planning is a fundamental aspect of diabetes management, offering several benefits for individuals with diabetes:

1. **Blood Sugar Control:**
   - Enables the creation of well-balanced meals, helping control blood sugar levels and reducing the risk of sudden spikes or crashes.

2. **Portion Control:**
   - Facilitates portion control, aiding in managing calorie intake and supporting weight management, a crucial aspect for individuals with diabetes.

3. **Balanced Nutrition:**
   - Ensures a balanced distribution of carbohydrates, proteins, and fats, providing essential nutrients for overall health.

4. **Consistency:**
   - Establishes a consistent eating pattern, which is vital for individuals with diabetes who often benefit from regular meals and snacks.

5. **Prevention of Impulse Eating:**
   - Reduces the likelihood of making unhealthy food choices on impulse, contributing to better adherence to dietary recommendations.

6. **Time-Efficiency:**
   - Saves time by reducing last-minute decisions about what to eat, making it easier to adhere to a healthy eating routine.

7. **Variety and Enjoyment:**
   - Allows for the inclusion of a variety of foods, promoting a diverse and enjoyable diet while meeting nutritional needs.

8. **Adaptability:**
   - Enables adjustments based on lifestyle, medication, and activity levels, providing a flexible approach to diabetes management.

Batch Cooking for Convenience

Batch cooking is a practical strategy that brings added convenience to meal planning for individuals with diabetes:

1. **Time Savings:**
   - Reduces the time spent on daily meal preparation by cooking larger quantities of food at once.

2. Consistent Portions:

   - Facilitates portion control as meals can be divided into appropriate serving sizes and stored for future consumption.

3. Minimizes Food Waste:

   - Helps minimize food waste by utilizing ingredients efficiently and preventing unused items from expiring.

4. Stress Reduction:

   - Alleviates stress associated with daily meal preparation, especially during busy times or when energy levels may be lower.

5. Nutrient Retention:

   - Preserves nutrient content as foods are cooked in larger batches, reducing exposure to heat and potential nutrient loss.

6. Diverse Meal Options:

   - Allows for the creation of diverse meals by combining batch-cooked components in various ways, adding variety to the diet.

7. Enhances Meal Variety:

   - Promotes a more varied diet by having a range of pre-prepared options available, reducing the monotony of daily meal choices.

Smart Grocery Shopping for Diabetic-Friendly Ingredients

Smart grocery shopping, combined with effective meal planning and batch cooking, lays the foundation for a balanced and diabetic-friendly eating routine. It empowers individuals with diabetes to make informed choices that support overall health and blood sugar management:

1. **Fresh Produce:**
   - Prioritize fresh fruits and vegetables, opting for a colorful variety to ensure a range of nutrients and fiber.

2. **Whole Grains:**
   - Choose whole grains such as brown rice, quinoa, oats, and whole wheat products for complex carbohydrates and added fiber.

3. **Lean Proteins:**
   - Select lean protein sources, including poultry, fish, tofu, legumes, and low-fat dairy, to support muscle health and blood sugar control.

4. **Healthy Fats:**
   - Include sources of healthy fats such as avocados, nuts, seeds, and olive oil for heart health and satiety.

5. **Low-Glycemic Index Foods:**
   - Incorporate low-GI foods, such as lentils, beans, and non-starchy vegetables, to help manage blood sugar levels.

6. **Dairy or Dairy Alternatives:**
   - Choose low-fat or non-fat dairy products or suitable alternatives to limit saturated fat intake.

7. **Limit Processed Foods:**
   - Minimize processed and sugary foods, opting for whole, minimally processed options to reduce added sugars and unhealthy fats.

8. **Read Nutrition Labels:**
   - Read nutrition labels to understand the composition of packaged foods, paying attention to carbohydrate content, fiber, and serving sizes.

9. **Plan Ahead:**
   - Create a shopping list based on planned meals, preventing impulse purchases and ensuring you have the necessary ingredients for diabetic-friendly meals.

10. **Hydration:**
    - Include water and other low-calorie, sugar-free beverages to stay hydrated without adding excess calories.

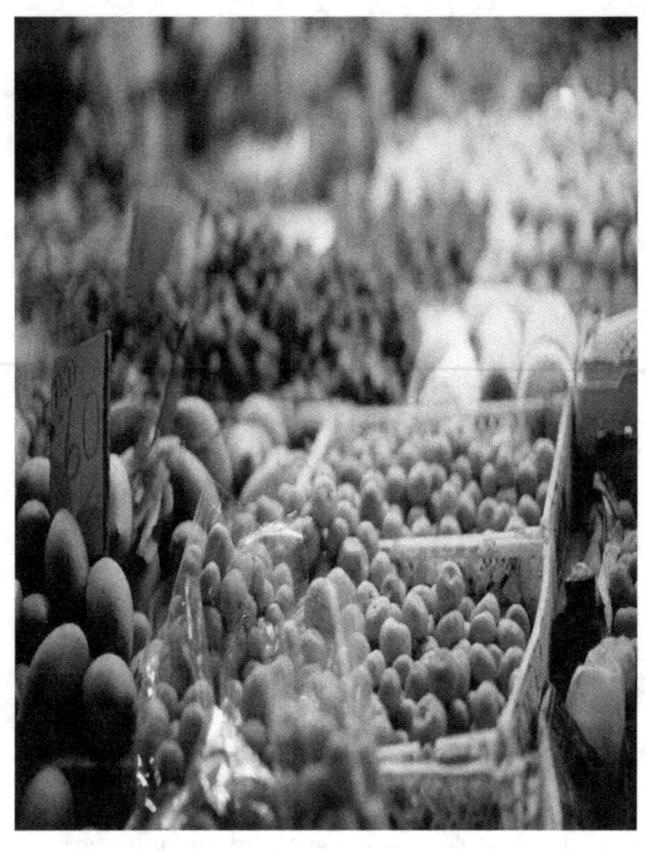

CHAPTER SIX

Delicious and Nutritious Recipes

Breakfast Ideas

1. **Greek Yogurt Parfait:**
   - Layer non-fat Greek yogurt with fresh berries, a sprinkle of chia seeds, and a drizzle of sugar-free honey.

2. **Vegetable Omelette:**
   - Whip up an omelette with egg whites, spinach, tomatoes, and a touch of feta cheese for a protein-packed and low-carb breakfast.

Lunch and Dinner Recipes

Lunch:

1.**Quinoa Salad with Avocado:**
   - Combine cooked quinoa with diced cucumber, cherry tomatoes, avocado, and grilled chicken. Dress with a lemon vinaigrette.

2. **Salmon Lettuce Wraps:**
   - Wrap grilled salmon in butter lettuce leaves, add sliced cucumber, avocado, and a dollop of Greek yogurt sauce.

Dinner:
1. **Zucchini Noodles with Pesto Chicken:**
   - Spiralize zucchini into noodles and top with grilled pesto chicken for a low-carb alternative to pasta.

2. **Turkey and Vegetable Stir-Fry:**
   - Stir-fry lean ground turkey with colorful vegetables like bell peppers, broccoli, and snap peas. Serve over cauliflower rice.

Snack and Dessert

Snack:
1.**Cottage Cheese and Berries:**
   - Pair low-fat cottage cheese with a mix of fresh berries for a satisfying and protein-rich snack.

2. **Spiced Roasted Chickpeas:**
   - Toss chickpeas with olive oil and spices, then roast until crispy. A crunchy and fiber-packed snack.

Dessert:
1.**Baked Cinnamon Apple Slices:**
   - Slice apples, sprinkle with cinnamon, and bake until tender. Top with a dollop of unsweetened Greek yogurt.

2. **Dark Chocolate-Dipped Strawberries:**
   - Dip fresh strawberries in melted dark chocolate for a delicious and antioxidant-rich dessert.

Bonus Treat:
1. **Chia Seed Pudding:**
   - Mix chia seeds with almond milk and let it sit overnight. Top with sliced almonds, berries, and a drizzle of sugar-free syrup.

2.**Veggie and Hummus Stuffed Peppers:**
   - Stuff mini bell peppers with hummus and assorted veggies for a crunchy and satisfying snack.

A Comprehensive Meal Plan

This plan includes breakfast, snacks, lunch, snacks, and dinner for each day.

Day	Breakfast	Lunch	Dinner	Snack
1	Scrambled eggs with spinach and whole-grain toast	Grilled chicken salad with vinaigrette	Baked salmon, quinoa, and asparagus	Greek yogurt with berries

Day	Breakfast	Lunch	Dinner	Snack
2	Oatmeal with sliced strawberries and almonds	Turkey and vegetable stir-fry with brown rice	Lentil soup with a side salad	Apple slices with peanut butter
3	Whole-grain pancakes with blueberries	Tofu and vegetable curry with quinoa	Grilled shrimp, broccoli, and sweet potato	Cottage cheese with pineapple chunks
4	Greek yogurt parfait with granola and mixed berries	Spinach and feta omelette with whole-grain toast	Baked cod with roasted Brussels sprouts	Handful of walnuts
5	Spinach and feta omelette, whole-grain toast	Veggie and hummus wrap with whole-grain tortilla	Grilled fish, quinoa, asparagus	Carrot sticks with hummus
6	Smoothie with spinach, berries, protein powder	Lentil and vegetable stir-fry with brown rice	Chicken Caesar salad with whole-grain croutons	Greek yogurt with almonds
7	Avocado toast on whole-grain bread	Turkey and vegetable skewers with quinoa	Baked cod, sweet potato wedges, steamed broccoli	Sliced cucumber with tzatziki

8	Chia seed pudding with mixed berries	Tofu and vegetable curry with brown rice	Grilled chicken, quinoa, roasted Brussels sprouts	Carrot and celery sticks with hummus
9	Whole-grain waffles with sliced banana	Chickpea salad with tomatoes and cucumbers	Baked salmon, quinoa, asparagus	Handful of walnuts
10	Scrambled eggs with mushrooms, whole-grain toast	Chicken Caesar wrap with whole-grain tortilla	Stir-fried shrimp with mixed vegetables, brown rice	Cottage cheese with pineapple chunks

Continue this pattern, adjusting based on preferences and nutritional needs, and ensuring a balance of lean proteins, whole grains, vegetables, and healthy fats. Adjust portion sizes based on individual needs and preferences.

Additional Tips:
- Incorporate a variety of vegetables, lean proteins, and whole grains.
- Monitor portion sizes and spread meals throughout the day.
- Stay hydrated with water or herbal teas.
- Limit added sugars and processed foods.
- Adjust the plan based on individual preferences and nutritional needs.

- Regularly monitor blood sugar levels.
- Consult healthcare professionals or dietitians for personalized advice.

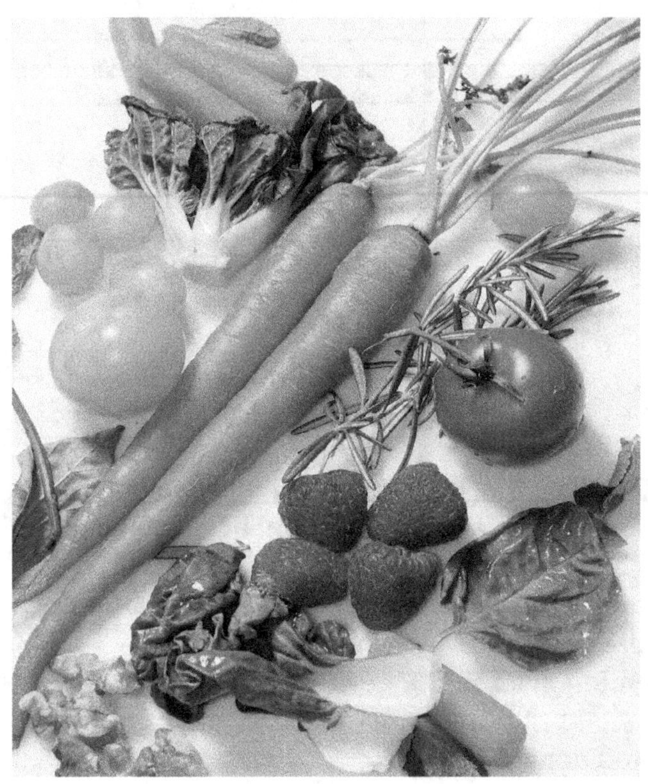

CHAPTER SEVEN

Eating Out and Social Situations

Making Wise Choices at Restaurants

Making wise food choices at restaurants is crucial for individuals with diabetes to maintain blood sugar control. It is essential to note that every restaurant is different, so these guidelines may need to be adapted based on the specific menu and cuisine. It's also beneficial to communicate with restaurant staff about your dietary needs to ensure a more tailored dining experience.
Guide to help you navigate restaurant menus:

1. **Review the Menu in Advance:**
   - Check online the restaurant's menu before going. This allows you to plan ahead and make informed choices.

2. **Choose Lean Proteins:**
   - Opt for grilled or baked lean proteins such as chicken, turkey, fish, or tofu. Avoid fried and breaded options.

3. **Select Whole Grains:**
   - Choose whole grains like brown rice, quinoa, or whole wheat options when available. Avoid refined grains like white rice or pasta.

4. **Load Up on Vegetables:**
   - Include a variety of non-starchy vegetables in your meal. These can be steamed, grilled, or in salads.

5. **Control Portion Sizes:**
   - Be mindful of portion sizes, and consider sharing large dishes or taking leftovers home.

6. **Ask for Modifications:**
   - Don't hesitate to ask for modifications to suit your dietary needs, such as dressing on the side, or steamed instead of fried.

7. **Limit Added Sugars:**
   - Choose dishes with minimal added sugars. Be cautious with sauces, dressings, and condiments that may contain hidden sugars.

8. **Watch for Hidden Fats:**
   - Be aware of hidden fats in dishes. Opt for grilled or baked options and request sauces or dressings on the side.

9. **Beverage Choices:**
   - Choose water, unsweetened tea, or black coffee instead of sugary drinks. If you consume alcohol, be mindful of your intake and be aware of its impact on blood sugar.

10. **Be Mindful of Appetizers:**
   - Consider healthier appetizers like a salad or vegetable-based dish. Skip fried options or those high in refined carbohydrates.

11. **Avoid All-You-Can-Eat Buffets:**
   - Buffets can make portion control challenging. If you choose a buffet, focus on smaller portions and a variety of nutrient-dense foods.

12. **Ask for Nutrition Information:**
   - Some restaurants provide nutritional information upon request. Use this information to make more informed choices.

13. **Plan for Dessert:**
   - If you want dessert, consider sharing with others at the table. Choose fruit-based options or those with controlled portion sizes.

14. **Stay Hydrated:**
   - Take water throughout the meal to stay hydrated and help control appetite.

15. **Listen to Your Body:**
   - Pay attention to hunger and fullness cues. Stop eating when satisfied, and avoid overindulging.

Navigating Social Events with Diabetes

Navigating social events with a diabetic-friendly diet requires planning and awareness. The strategies to help you maintain blood sugar control during such situations are:

1. **Communicate Dietary Needs:**
   - Inform hosts or event organizers about your dietary restrictions. Most are willing to accommodate special requests.

2. **Eat Before You Go:**
   - Have a balanced meal or snack before attending the event. This can help you avoid excessive hunger and make better food choices.

3. **Choose Wisely:**
   - Survey the available food options before filling your plate. Go for lean proteins, vegetables, and whole grains when possible.

4. **Control Portions:**
   - Be mindful of portion sizes, especially with high-carbohydrate or sugary foods. Use smaller plates if available.

5. **Limit Alcohol Intake:**
   - If you consume alcohol, do so in moderation. Alcohol can affect blood sugar levels, so monitor and adjust accordingly.

6. **Stay Active:**
   - Engage in social activities that involve movement, such as dancing or taking a walk. Physical activity helps regulate blood sugar.

7. **Plan for Desserts:**
   - If you want dessert, consider sharing or choosing a smaller portion. Opt for fruit-based or lower-sugar options when available.

8. **Bring a Dish:**
   - Offer to bring a diabetic-friendly dish to share. This ensures there's at least one option that aligns with your dietary needs.

Tips for Traveling with a Diabetic-Friendly Diet

1. **Pack Snacks:**
   - Bring diabetic-friendly snacks like nuts, seeds, whole fruit, or cut veggies to have on hand. This helps control hunger and prevents impulsive food choices.

2. **Research Local Cuisine:**
   - Research the local cuisine and identify diabetic-friendly options at your travel destination. This knowledge can guide your food choices.

3. **Inform Travel Companions:**
   - Inform travel companions about your dietary needs so they can support your choices and help plan meals.

4. **Carry Medications and Supplies:**
   - Pack enough medications, testing supplies, and snacks for the duration of your trip. Keep them easily accessible, especially if you're flying.

5. **Stay Hydrated:**
   - Drink plenty of water, especially if traveling by air. Dehydration can affect blood sugar levels, so stay well-hydrated.

6. **Choose Smartly at Restaurants:**
   - When dining out, choose restaurants that offer healthy options. Ask for modifications if needed, and be cautious with portion sizes.

7. **Time Your Meals:**
   - Stick to a regular meal schedule as much as possible, even in different time zones. Consistency helps regulate blood sugar levels.

8. **Be Prepared for Emergencies:**
   - Carry a list of emergency contacts, your doctor's information, and details about your diabetes management plan.

9. **Consider Travel Insurance:**

- Consider travel insurance that includes medical emergencies. It guarantees peace of mind in case unexpected health issues arise.

10. **Adapt to Local Ingredients:**

- Be flexible and adapt your meals based on the availability of local ingredients. Embrace new, healthy options.

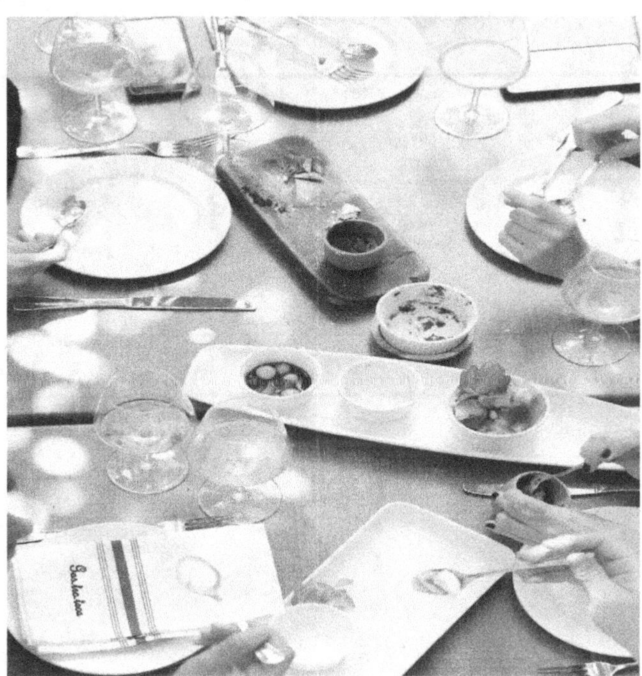

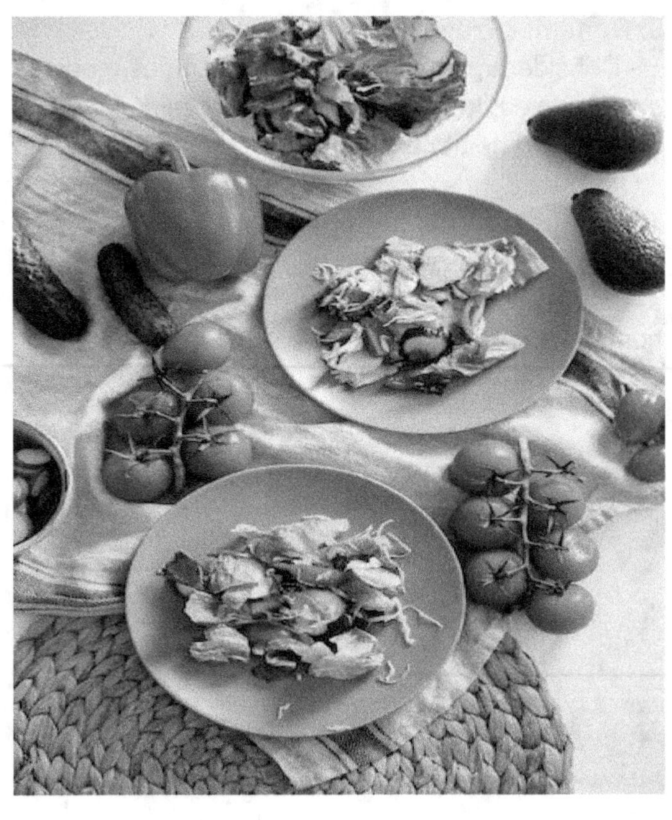

CHAPTER 8

Exercise and Physical Activity

Tailoring Exercise for Diabetics

Exercise is beneficial for individuals with diabetes, helping to improve blood sugar control, enhance insulin sensitivity, and promote overall health. Remember, individual responses to exercise can vary, so it's crucial to listen to your body and make adjustments as needed. Let's review some exercise recommendations for individuals with diabetes:

1. **Consult with Healthcare Professionals:**
   - Before starting a new exercise program, consult with your healthcare team, including your doctor and a qualified fitness professional for personalized advice based on your specific health condition.
2. **Aerobic Exercise:**
   - Engage in moderate-intensity aerobic exercise for at least 150 minutes per week, spread across most days. This can include brisk walking, cycling, swimming, or dancing. For greater benefits, aim for 300 minutes of aerobic exercise per week.

3. **Strength Training:**
   - Include strength training exercises at least two days per week. Focus on major muscle groups, incorporating exercises such as weight lifting, resistance band workouts, or bodyweight exercises.

4. **Flexibility and Balance Training:**

   - Incorporate flexibility and balance exercises into your routine. Activities like yoga or tai chi can help improve flexibility, balance, and reduce the risk of falls.

5. **Interval Training:**

   - Consider interval training, alternating between higher and lower-intensity exercise. This approach can be effective in managing blood sugar levels.

6. **Regular Physical Activity:**

   - Aim for daily physical activity. Short bouts of exercise throughout the day can be as beneficial as continuous sessions. Find opportunities to move, such as taking the stairs or going for a short walk.

7. **Individualized Approach:**

   - Channel your exercise plan to your fitness level, health status, and personal preferences. This ensures sustainability and enjoyment, increasing the likelihood of adherence.

8. **Monitor Blood Sugar Levels:**

   - Constantly monitor your blood sugar levels, especially before and after exercise. This helps you understand how different activities affect your body, allowing for adjustments in your management plan.

9. **Stay Hydrated:**
   - Take water before, during, and after exercise to stay hydrated. Dehydration can affect blood sugar levels, so it's essential to maintain proper fluid balance.

10. **Choose Safe Activities:**
    - Select activities that are safe and suitable for your health condition. Avoid exercises that may cause injury or complications.

11. **Wear Appropriate Footwear:**
    - Wear comfortable and supportive footwear, especially if you have diabetic neuropathy. Check your feet regularly for any signs of injury or discomfort.

12. **Consider Weather Conditions:**
    - Be mindful of extreme weather conditions, especially if exercising outdoors. Adjust your activities accordingly to ensure safety and comfort.

13. **Integrate Physical Activity into Daily Life:**
    - Look for opportunities to be active throughout the day, such as gardening, house chores, or taking breaks to stretch at work.

14. **Emergency Preparedness:**
    - If you're exercising alone, let someone know your plans, carry identification, and be aware of the signs of hypoglycemia (low blood sugar) to respond promptly if needed.

15. **Enjoyment and Variety:**
   - Select activities you enjoy to make exercise a positive and sustainable part of your routine. Incorporate variety to prevent boredom and target different muscle groups.

Combining Diet and Exercise for Weight Loss

Effective weight loss is achieved through a synergistic combination of a balanced diet and regular exercise. The combination of a healthy diet and regular exercise not only aids weight loss but also promotes overall well-being and sustainable lifestyle changes:

1. **Balanced Diet:**
   - Maintain whole, nutrient-dense foods like fruits, vegetables, lean proteins, and whole grains.
   - Control portion sizes to manage calorie intake.
   - Be mindful of added sugars and processed foods, opting for natural and unprocessed alternatives.

2. **Caloric Deficit:**
   - Create a caloric deficit by consuming fewer calories than your body expends.

3. **Meal Timing:**
   - Consider spreading meals throughout the day to maintain energy levels and prevent overeating.

Include a mix of macronutrients for sustained energy.

4. **Hydration:**
   - Stay adequately hydrated, as water can help control appetite and support metabolic processes. Limit sugary drinks and prioritize water.

5. **Regular Exercise:**
   - Combine aerobic exercises (e.g., walking, jogging) for calorie burning with strength training to build lean muscle, boosting metabolism.
   - Aim for at least 150 minutes of moderate-intensity aerobic exercise per week, along with muscle-strengthening activities on two or more days.

6. **Consistency and Patience:**
   - Establish sustainable habits. Consistency is crucial for long-term success.
   - Understand that weight loss takes time; set realistic goals and focus on overall health improvement.

7. **Individualized Approach:**
   - Customize your plan based on personal preferences, fitness levels, and any existing health conditions.
   - Consult with healthcare or fitness professionals for guidance tailored to your specific needs.

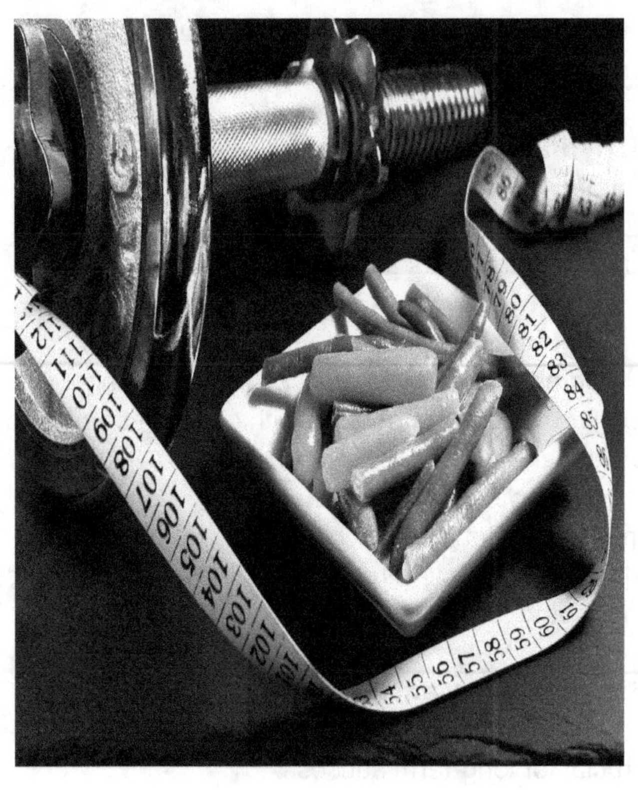

CHAPTER 9

Managing Stress and Sleep

Impact of Stress on Blood Sugar

Effectively managing stress contributes to better blood sugar control and overall diabetes management.Here's how stress affects blood sugar:

1. **Hormonal Response:**
   - Stress stimulates the release of stress hormones like cortisol and adrenaline.
   - These hormones can raise blood sugar levels by advancing the release of glucose from the liver.

2. **Insulin Resistance:**
   - Chronic stress may contribute to insulin resistance, where cells become less responsive to insulin.
   - This can hinder the body's ability to regulate blood sugar effectively.

3. **Changes in Eating Habits:**
   - Stress can lead to emotional eating or changes in eating habits.
   - Individuals may choose comfort foods high in sugar and carbohydrates, affecting blood sugar levels.

4. **Physical Activity Impact:**

   - Stress may lead to a decrease in physical activity, which can affect blood sugar regulation.

   - Regular exercise helps manage stress and can improve insulin sensitivity.

5. **Medication Effects:**

   - Stress can influence adherence to medication regimens.

   - Failure to adhere to prescribed medications may result in blood sugar fluctuations.

6. **Individual Variability:**

   - Responses to stress vary among individuals. Some may experience elevated blood sugar, while others may see a decrease.

Managing stress is crucial for individuals with diabetes. Strategies include:

- **Stress Reduction Techniques:**

   - Incorporate stress-relieving activities such as deep breathing, meditation, yoga, or regular exercise.

- **Consistent Blood Sugar Monitoring:**

   - Monitor blood sugar levels regularly, especially during stressful periods.

- **Healthy Lifestyle Choices:**

   - Maintain a balanced diet, regular exercise, and adequate sleep to support overall well-being.

- **Seeking Support:**
  - Engage with healthcare professionals or support networks to address stress-related concerns and find appropriate coping strategies.

Importance of Adequate Sleep for Weight Management

For individuals with diabetes, ensuring adequate sleep is particularly crucial for effective weight management due to the intricate relationship between sleep, hormones, and blood sugar regulation:

1. **Blood Sugar Control:**
   - Sufficient sleep is linked to better insulin sensitivity, helping to regulate blood sugar levels effectively.
   - Lack of sleep may lead to insulin resistance, contributing to elevated blood sugar levels, a significant concern for those with diabetes.

2. **Hormonal Balance:**
   - Quality sleep influences hormones involved in appetite and metabolism, such as ghrelin and leptin.
   - Disruptions in sleep patterns can lead to increased ghrelin (appetite stimulant) and decreased leptin (satiety hormone), potentially impacting food choices and intake.

3. Stress Management:

   - Adequate sleep plays a vital role in managing stress, as sleep deprivation can elevate cortisol levels.
   - Elevated cortisol levels may contribute to insulin resistance and hinder optimal blood sugar control.

4. Promoting Healthy Lifestyle Choices:

   - A well-rested individual is more likely to engage in physical activity and make healthier food choices, essential components of diabetes management and weight control.

5. Consistency in Routine:

   - Establishing a regular sleep routine helps maintain consistency in circadian rhythms, supporting metabolic health and blood sugar regulation.

6. Reducing Cravings:

   - Quality sleep helps regulate the brain's reward centers, reducing cravings for unhealthy, high-calorie foods.
   - Improved sleep can contribute to better adherence to a diabetic-friendly diet.

To prioritize sleep for effective weight management with diabetes:
- Aim for 7-9 hours of sleep per night.
- Maintain a consistent sleep schedule, even on weekends.

- Create a conducive sleep environment,
minimizing disruptions.
- Manage stress through relaxation techniques.

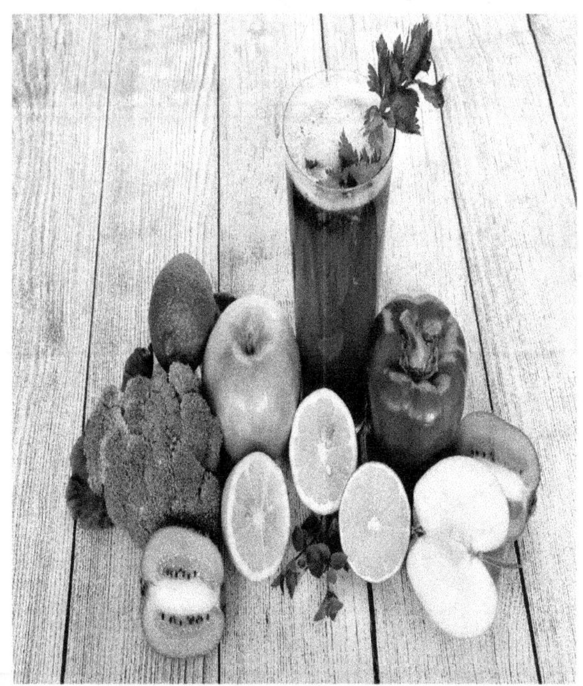

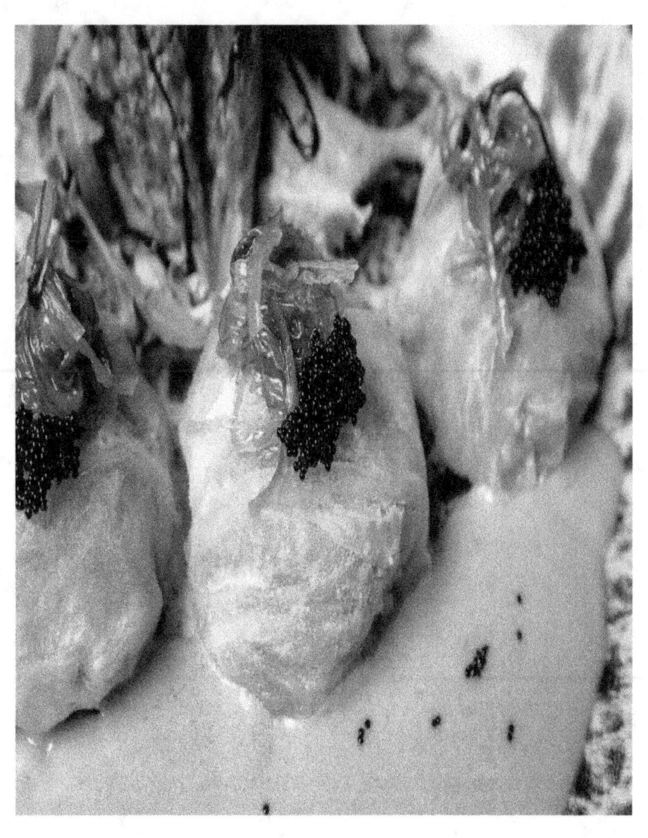

Chapter 10

Monitoring Blood Sugar Levels

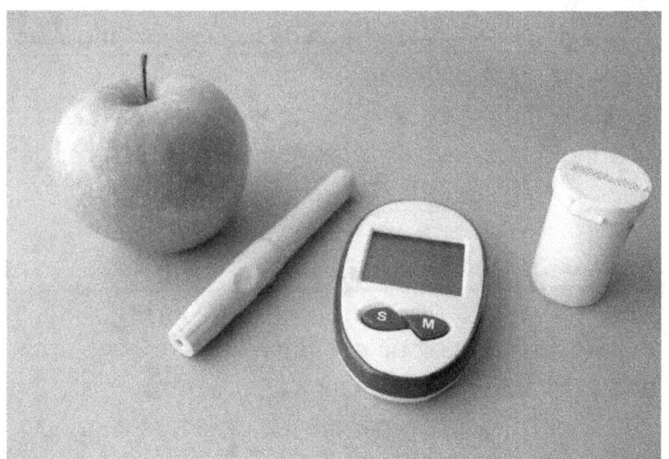

Regular Monitoring Techniques

Empowering individuals with diabetes through regular monitoring techniques ensures they have the tools and knowledge to make informed decisions about their health. Regular monitoring is a key element in the proactive management of diabetes. Here are diabetic-friendly techniques for regular monitoring:

1. Glucometers:
   - Explain the proper use of glucometers for at-home blood sugar testing.

- Emphasize the importance of clean hands and proper storage of test strips to ensure accurate readings.

2. Continuous Glucose Monitoring (CGM) Systems:

- Introduce CGM systems as a convenient option for real-time monitoring.
- Highlight the benefits of continuous tracking, offering a more comprehensive view of blood sugar trends.

3. Newer Technologies:

- Discuss advancements in blood sugar monitoring technologies, such as smartphone apps and wearable devices.
- Emphasize user-friendly features for those who may be less tech-savvy.

4. Self-Monitoring Education:

- Provide education on interpreting blood sugar readings and understanding target ranges.
- Encourage individuals to become familiar with their own baseline readings and to recognize patterns.

5. Post-Meal Readings:

- Stress the importance of post-meal readings to assess the impact of different foods on blood sugar levels.
- Offer guidance on optimal timing for post-meal testing.

6. Trend Analysis:
   - Guide individuals on analyzing trends and patterns in their blood sugar readings.
   - Encourage tracking factors such as physical activity, stress levels, and medication adjustments to identify correlations.

7. Portable Monitoring for On-the-Go:
   - Discuss portable monitoring options for individuals with active lifestyles.
   - Explore compact devices and accessories that make on-the-go monitoring more convenient.

8. User-Friendly Resources:
   - Recommend user-friendly resources, such as mobile apps with features like data visualization and medication reminders.
   - Highlight the importance of regularly updating and syncing devices for accurate data.

Adjusting Meal Plans Based on Blood Sugar Readings

Empowering individuals with diabetes to adjust their meal plans based on blood sugar readings fosters proactive and personalized management. A guide on adjusting meal plans for optimal blood sugar control:

1. Interpreting Blood Sugar Readings:

   - Explain target blood sugar ranges for fasting, pre-meal, and post-meal readings.

   - Emphasize the significance of understanding individualized target ranges based on healthcare provider recommendations.

2. Portion Control:

   - Discuss the impact of portion sizes on blood sugar levels.

   - Provide practical tips for portion control, such as using smaller plates and measuring serving sizes.

3. Carbohydrate Counting:

   - Educate on carbohydrate counting to help manage post-meal blood sugar levels.

   - Provide resources for identifying and calculating the carbohydrate content of different foods.

4. Low Glycemic Index Foods:

   - Highlight the benefits of incorporating low glycemic index foods, which have a slower impact on blood sugar, into meal plans.

   - Offer a list of diabetic-friendly foods with lower glycemic index values.

5. Balanced Meal Composition:

   - Emphasize the importance of a balanced meal composition, including proteins, fats, and fiber alongside carbohydrates.

   - Guide on creating well-rounded meals that contribute to stable blood sugar levels.

6. Timing of Meals:

- Discuss the impact of meal timing on blood sugar regulation.
- Encourage consistent meal schedules and avoiding prolonged periods between meals.

7. Post-Meal Adjustments:

- Explain strategies for adjusting subsequent meals based on post-meal blood sugar readings.
- Provide examples of making modifications to prevent large fluctuations.

8. Collaboration with Healthcare Professionals:

- Stress the importance of regular communication with healthcare providers regarding blood sugar readings and meal plan adjustments.
- Encourage individuals to seek guidance on modifying meal plans in response to changing health needs.

9. Personalized Approaches:

- Acknowledge the uniqueness of each individual's response to foods and medications.
- Encourage a personalized approach to meal planning, considering lifestyle, preferences, and health goals.

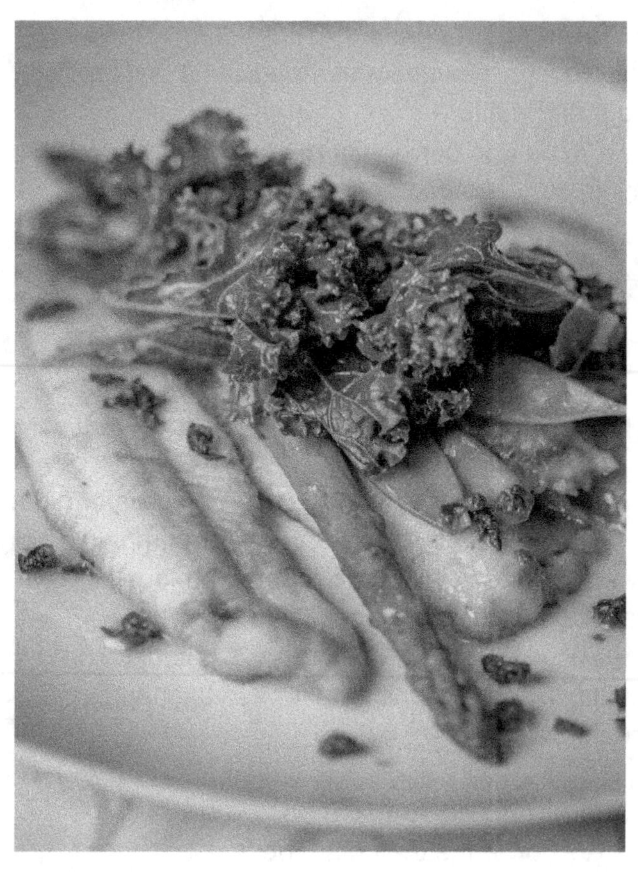

CHAPTER ELEVEN

Celebrating Successes and Overcoming Challenges

In the journey of diabetes management, acknowledging successes and addressing challenges is vital for long-term well-being. This chapter explores strategies for staying motivated and overcoming common challenges.

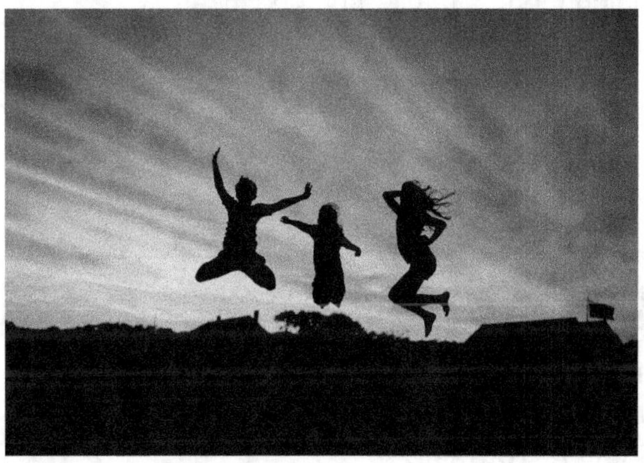

Staying Motivated

1. **Celebrate Small Wins:**
   - Acknowledge and celebrate small achievements in blood sugar control and healthy habits. Each success is a step towards long-term well-being.

2. **Visualize Health Goals:**
   - Create a clear picture of your health goals. Visualizing the positive outcomes can serve as a powerful motivator, reinforcing the significance of your efforts.

3. **Set Realistic and Achievable Goals:**
   - Establish goals that are realistic and attainable. This makes the journey more manageable and builds confidence as you achieve each milestone.

4. **Establish a Support System:**
   - Surround yourself with a supportive network, including friends, family, and healthcare professionals. Sharing your journey with others provides encouragement and understanding.

5. **Find Joy in the Process:**
   - Discover enjoyment in adopting a healthier lifestyle. Whether it's trying new recipes, exploring different forms of exercise, or practicing mindfulness, finding joy in the process enhances motivation.

6. **Educate Yourself:**
   - Continuously educate yourself about diabetes management. Understanding the impact of your choices on your health fosters a sense of empowerment and responsibility.

7. **Focus on Overall Well-Being:**
   - Shift the focus from solely controlling diabetes to enhancing overall well-being. When you prioritize holistic health, managing diabetes becomes a part of a broader commitment to a healthier lifestyle.

8. **Reward Yourself Without Food:**
   - Celebrate achievements with non-food rewards. Treat yourself to activities or items that bring joy, reinforcing positive behaviors without compromising your health.

9. **Track Progress:**
   - Keep a record of your progress. Tracking improvements in blood sugar levels, lifestyle changes, and overall health serves as a tangible reminder of your achievements.

10. **Reflect on Motivations:**
    - Regularly reflect on why diabetes control is important to you. Connecting with your deeper motivations strengthens your resolve during challenging times.

11. **Embrace Flexibility:**
    - Understand that setbacks are a natural part of any journey. Embrace flexibility and view challenges as opportunities to learn and adjust your approach.

12. **Celebrate Personal Growth:**
   - Recognize the personal growth that comes from managing diabetes. The resilience and discipline developed through this journey contribute to your overall character and well-being.

Remember, sustaining efforts to control diabetes is a continuous journey. Stay motivated by focusing on the positive aspects, finding joy in the process, and celebrating both the small and significant victories along the way.

Addressing Common Challenges

By addressing these common challenges with a proactive and personalized approach, individuals managing diabetes and weight loss can enhance their overall well-being and achieve sustainable success.

1. **Meal Planning and Timing:**
   - Challenge: Balancing blood sugar while managing calorie intake can be complex.
   - **Solution:** Work with a dietitian to create a personalized meal plan that considers both nutritional needs and weight loss goals. Focus on consistent meal timing and portion control.

2. Physical Activity:

- **Challenge:** Finding enjoyable and sustainable exercises that accommodate individual fitness levels.

- **Solution:** Explore various activities and choose those you enjoy. Gradually increase intensity and duration, aiming for a mix of aerobic and strength training exercises.

3. Medication Adjustments:

- **Challenge:** Fluctuations in blood sugar levels may require adjustments to medication, impacting weight.

- **Solution:** Regularly communicate with healthcare professionals. They can tailor medication regimens to support both blood sugar control and weight management.

4. Emotional Eating:

- **Challenge:** Coping with stress or emotions through unhealthy eating habits.

- **Solution:** Develop alternative coping mechanisms, such as mindfulness, meditation, or engaging in hobbies.

5. Social and Cultural Influences:

- **Challenge:** Navigating social situations and cultural expectations around food choices.

- **Solution:** Communicate dietary needs with others and explore healthier alternatives that align with cultural preferences. Plan ahead for social events to make informed choices.

6. **Plateaus and Setbacks:**
   - **Challenge:** Experiencing plateaus in weight loss or setbacks in blood sugar control.
   - **Solution:** View setbacks as learning opportunities. Adjust your approach, seek guidance from healthcare professionals, and stay committed to long-term goals.

7. **Time Management:**
   - **Challenge:** Balancing work, family, and self-care responsibilities.
   - **Solution:** Prioritize self-care and plan meals and exercise routines in advance. Break down goals into smaller, manageable tasks to fit into a busy schedule.

8. **Support System:**
   - **Challenge:** Lack of a supportive network or understanding from those around you.
   - **Solution:** Educate your support system about your journey and involve them in your efforts. Seek encouragement from diabetes support groups or online communities.

9. **Body Image Concerns:**
   - **Challenge:** Navigating changes in body composition and dealing with body image concerns.
   - **Solution:** Focus on overall health and well-being rather than just weight loss. Celebrate achievements beyond physical appearance and prioritize self-acceptance.

10. **Consistency:**
   - **Challenge:** Maintaining consistent lifestyle changes over time.
   - **Solution:** Set realistic and achievable goals. Foster a mindset of gradual progress and adaptability. Celebrate both short-term and long-term successes to stay motivated.

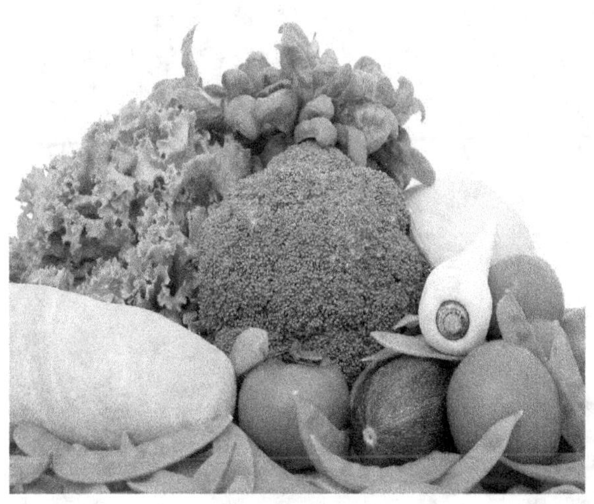

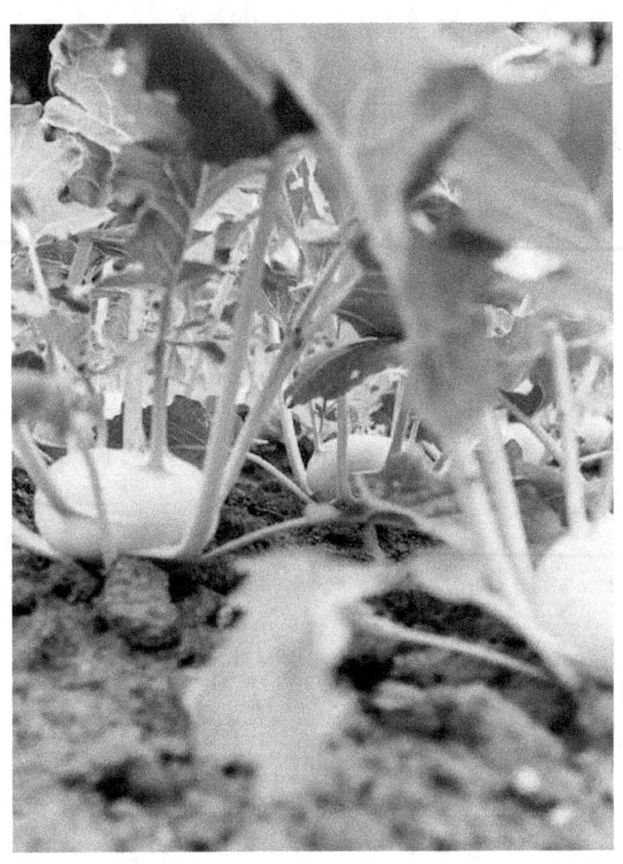

CONCLUSION

In drawing the final threads together on the intricate tapestry of diabetic-friendly meal plans for weight loss, it becomes evident that this approach is not merely about shedding pounds but is a holistic journey toward enhanced well-being and effective diabetes management.

Key Points Recap

1. Balanced Nutrition as a Foundation:

 - Diabetic-friendly meal plans emphasize a balanced intake of carbohydrates, proteins, and healthy fats, underlining the importance of comprehensive nutrition for sustainable health.

2. Mindful Carbohydrate Management:

 - Understanding the impact of carbohydrates on blood sugar levels is crucial. Meal plans incorporate mindful carbohydrate choices, focusing on quality, portion control, and considering the glycemic index.

3. Inclusion of Nutrient-Dense Foods:

 - Prioritizing nutrient-dense foods rich in vitamins, minerals, and antioxidants ensures that the body receives essential nutrients while managing calorie intake.

4. Portion Control for Caloric Management:

 - Portion control emerges as a guiding principle, not only for weight regulation but also for maintaining stable blood sugar levels, contributing to a harmonious approach to diabetes management.

5. *Protein and Healthy Fats for Satiety:*
   - Incorporating lean proteins and healthy fats fosters a sense of satiety, contributing not only to weight loss goals but also to overall metabolic health.

6. *Regular Monitoring for Informed Choices:*
   - Regular blood sugar monitoring provides valuable insights, allowing individuals to make informed choices, adapt their meal plans, and maintain stability in blood sugar levels.

7. *Synergy with Physical Activity:*
   - Diabetic-friendly meal plans complement regular exercise, creating a synergy that promotes weight loss, improves insulin sensitivity, and enhances overall physical well-being.

8. *Individualized Approaches for Long-Term Success:*
   - Acknowledging the uniqueness of each individual, the emphasis on tailoring meal plans to personal preferences, lifestyle, and health needs fosters adherence and ensures long-term success.

Encouragement for Sustainable Lifestyle Changes

As we conclude this exploration, it's vital to recognize that diabetic-friendly meal plans for weight loss are not a temporary fix but a sustainable lifestyle shift. This journey is about more than numbers on a scale; it's about reclaiming control, fostering health, and finding joy in nourishing the body.

Every Meal, a Step Towards Wellness:
   - Each meal becomes an opportunity to fuel the body with intention, a step towards wellness, and a demonstration of self-care.

Adaptability and Resilience:
   - Recognize the adaptability and resilience within. This journey may have its challenges, but every challenge is a chance to learn, grow, and refine the approach to achieving health goals.

Celebrating Progress:
   - Celebrate not just the end goal but every step taken, every healthy choice made, and every positive change embraced. Progress is a journey, and every journey deserves acknowledgment.

Empowerment for Life:
   - Ultimately, diabetic-friendly meal plans for weight loss are an empowering strategy that transcends weight management. It is a commitment

to a lifestyle that not only fosters a healthy body but also nurtures a resilient spirit, paving the way for a life rich in vitality and well-being.

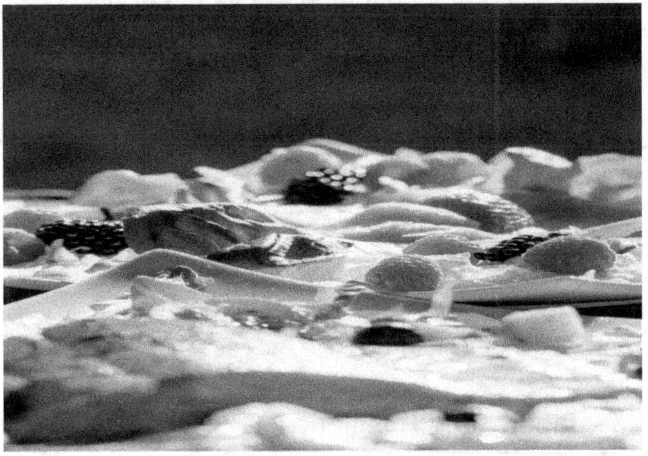

APPENDIX

Glossary of Terms

This glossary aims to provide clarity on key terms related to diabetes and nutrition, facilitating a better understanding of the principles involved in managing this condition.

1. **Diabetes Mellitus:**
   - A chronic medical condition characterized by elevated blood sugar levels due to insufficient insulin production or ineffective use of insulin.

2. **Insulin:**
   - A hormone produced by the pancreas that regulates blood sugar levels by facilitating the absorption of glucose into cells.

3. **Type 1 Diabetes:**
   - An autoimmune condition where the immune system attacks and destroys insulin-producing cells in the pancreas, leading to a lack of insulin production.

4. **Type 2 Diabetes:**
   - A condition characterized by insulin resistance, where the body's cells do not respond effectively to insulin, resulting in elevated blood sugar levels.

5. **Gestational Diabetes:**
   - Diabetes that develops during pregnancy and increases the risk of type 2 diabetes later in life.

6. **Blood Glucose:**
   - The concentration of glucose (sugar) present in the bloodstream.

7. **Hyperglycemia:**
   - Elevated blood sugar levels, a common feature of diabetes.

8. **Hypoglycemia:**
   - Abnormally low blood sugar levels, often caused by excessive insulin or insufficient food intake.

9. **Carbohydrates:**
   - One of the three main macronutrients, including sugars, starches, and fibers, which impact blood sugar levels.

10. **Glycemic Index (GI):**
   - A numerical scale indicating how quickly a carbohydrate-containing food raises blood sugar levels.

11. **Insulin Resistance:**
   - A condition where cells in the body do not respond properly to insulin, leading to elevated blood sugar levels.

12. A1c (Glycated Hemoglobin):

   - A blood test that measures average blood sugar levels over the past 2-3 months, providing an indication of long-term diabetes management.

13. Portion Control:

   - Managing the amount of food consumed to regulate calorie intake and control blood sugar levels.

14. Fiber:

   - A component of plant-based foods that aids digestion, helps control blood sugar, and promotes a feeling of fullness.

15. Nutrient-Dense Foods:

   - Foods that provide a high amount of nutrients relative to their calorie content.

16. Lean Proteins:

   - Protein sources that are low in saturated fats, such as poultry, fish, tofu, and legumes.

17. Glucometer:

   - A device used to measure blood sugar levels at home through a small drop of blood.

18. Continuous Glucose Monitoring (CGM):

   - A system that continuously tracks blood sugar levels throughout the day, providing real-time data to manage diabetes.

19. **Dietitian/Nutritionist:**
   - A healthcare professional specializing in nutrition who provides guidance on dietary choices, meal planning, and lifestyle changes.

20. **Mindful Eating:**
   - A practice involving paying attention to the present moment while eating, promoting awareness of hunger, fullness, and food choices.

Additional Resources

These additional resources offer a diverse range of information, from dietary guidelines and recipes to community support. Whether you're seeking expert advice, recipes, or peer support, these resources aim to empower individuals in managing diabetes through informed and healthy nutrition.

1. **Diabetes Care and Education (DCE) - Academy of Nutrition and Dietetics:**
   - Website: [DCE - Diabetes Care and Education](https://www.eatrightpro.org/practice/medicalnutrition-therapy/diabetes-care-and-education)

2. **American Heart Association - Diabetes and Heart-Healthy Meals:**
   - Website: [AHA - Diabetes and Heart-Healthy Meals](https://www.heart.org/en/health-topics/diabetes)

3. **Diabetes Self-Management:**
   - Website: [Diabetes Self-Management - Nutrition](https://www.diabetesselfmanagement.com/nutrition-exercise/nutrition/)

4. **Nutrition.gov - Diabetes Resources:**
   - Website: [Nutrition.gov - Diabetes Resources](https://www.nutrition.gov/subject/health/diabetes)

5. **Diabetes Forecast - Recipes:**
   - Website: [Diabetes Forecast - Recipes](https://www.diabetesforecast.org/landing-pages/lp-recipes.html)

6. **Beyond Type 1 - Nutrition and Recipes:**
   - Website: [Beyond Type 1 - Nutrition](https://beyondtype1.org/living-with-type-1/nutrition/)

7. **The Diabetic Chef's Year-Round Cookbook by Chris Smith:**
   - Book: [The Diabetic Chef's Year-Round Cookbook](https://www.amazon.com/Diabetic-Chefs-Year-Round-Cookbook/dp/1580400937)

8. **Diabetes UK - Enjoy Food:**
   - Website: [Diabetes UK - Enjoy Food](https://www.diabetes.org.uk/guide-to-diabetes/enjoy-food)

9. **Harvard Health Publishing - Diabetes and Nutrition:**
   - Website: [Harvard Health - Diabetes and Nutrition](https://www.health.harvard.edu/topics/diabetes-and-diet)

10. **TuDiabetes Forum:**
    - Online Community: [TuDiabetes Forum](https://forum.tudiabetes.org/)